The End

*Obesity does not just affect individuals; its impact is felt predominantly within the **family**, the backbone of society. The book cover reflects the above concept with an illustration of the basic family unit: mother, father, and children.*

The
END
of
OBESITY

Samuel N. Grief, MD
Sophie Ares-Grief, RD

G&G Publishing
379 Amherst St., Suite 202, Nashua, NH 03063

Note: This book is intended for general health care information only and not as a substitute for medical advice by a personal health care provider. Readers are urged to discuss their own health issues with a trusted health care provider before beginning any personal weight loss or exercise program.

All rights reserved. No part of this book may be reproduced or transmitted in any form or by any means, electronic or mechanical, including photocopying, recording, or by any information storage and retrieval system without prior written permission of the publisher.

Printed in the United States of America

ISBN (paperback): 0-9660563-0-2

Copyright © 1998 by Samuel N. Grief, MD

Dedication

This book is dedicated to our parents. Their unconditional love and lifelong encouragement have helped us to find our own unique paths in this world.

Table of Contents

Introduction..................................1

1 Seven Steps to Losing Weight 13
   and Keeping it Off
2 A Dietitian's Perspective 27
3 Time to Eat 47
4 Back to Basics: The Food Guide Pyramid 57
5 The Truth about Fats and Oils 69

The Miracle Foods: An Introduction........... 75
6 Eat Your Veggies! 79
7 An Apple a Day............................ 83
8 Vitamins and Minerals...................... 91

9 Mood for Food 105
10 At the Gym 121

Running with Dad........................... 139

11 At the Coffee Shop 143
12 At the Buffet 149
13 At the Restaurant........................ 163
14 Children and Obesity..................... 171
15 "Magic" Pills............................ 187
16 "Wonder" Diets 201

Your Turn 217
Recommended Reading 219

Acknowledgements

We would like to thank Joyce Griffith, our hard-working editor, in helping us publish this book. Her personal touch was greatly appreciated.

Preface

The idea for *The End of Obesity* came to me on a wet and rainy spring day some time ago when one of my patients offered this comment: "Dr. Sam, I am thankful for the help you and your wife have given me. However, it would be nice if I could refer to all of this useful health and nutrition advice when I need to." That waas the catalyst I needed to begin working on this book.

Writing this book has been a challenge of perseverance and commitment to both my own beliefs and my career. In my heart, writing as a career is now a close runner-up to medicine. The marriage of these two creative and fascinating professions may lead me to author or co-author many more books on topics that have touched my heart.

My true love in life, however, is my beautiful wife, Sophie. Her tireless work on this book has made *The End of Obesity* a book I am proud to call our own. Thank you, Sophie.

Introduction

What disease costs American taxpayers more than 70 billion dollars annually and is responsible for an ever-rising toll in sickness and death?

What disease has plagued all developed countries of the twentieth century and is now threatening to become the No. 1 worldwide epidemic of the twenty-first century?

What disease is a contributing factor to heart disease, cancer, stroke, diabetes, and many more all too common medical conditions?

What disease affects more than one third of all American adults, nearly 30 percent of all American adolescents, and is on the rise in all segments of our society, including our most precious resource, our children?

Finally, what disease is almost entirely preventable by changing the way we eat, sleep, and live our daily lives?

If you answered "obesity" to all of the above questions, you would be right. Obesity is the scourge of our modern-day living. It is the second leading cause of preventable death in the United States, surpassed only by the cigarette. Obesity is a rapidly growing problem. In 1980, 25 percent of the adult U.S. population was obese; in 1997 the rate of obesity is 33 percent of all American adults and is climbing!

As most of us are now frighteningly aware, obesity is directly related to most of our North American lifestyle diseases: heart disease and stroke, diabetes, high blood pressure, certain types of cancer (breast, prostate, for example), gout, degenerative joint disease, sleep apnea, gallstones, and many more.

The topic of obesity has probably generated more discussion, more books, more proposed cures, and more of our collective brain power than any other health-related topic. This seven-letter condition has clutched North America since the beginning of the twentieth century and fails to loosen its suffocating noose around our necks.

As human beings it is only natural for us to seek a simpler and quicker way to accomplish our tasks. When it comes to weight loss, Americans have been searching for the elusive "quick fix" to reach their ideal weight for decades. Millions of Americans attempt to lose excess body weight through a variety of weight loss programs. Commercial slim-down products and programs dominate the weight-loss industry. Americans spend an estimated $30 billion on dieting every year.

A recent player in the weight-loss market is the dietary supplement. Dietary supplements (also known as "nutritional supplements") include products such as vitamins, minerals, protein powders, herbal preparations, and more. Go to any pharmacy or supermarket in your neighborhood and you will find a growing shelf of dietary or nutritional supplements. These supplements comprise a large portion of our expanding American

INTRODUCTION

economy and will likely make up an even bigger share of the global economy as we enter a new century.

Why is it that over 58 million American adults in our highly civilized and developed society are subjugated by obesity? What makes this heavyweight villain the No. 1 nemesis of North Americans? Why have we not been able to overcome and conquer this human frailty of ours?

I submit to you that there is only one real reason why North Americans and the rest of the world's advanced societies have not yet been able to harness this out-of-control juggernaut called obesity. The answer is only one word, but the ramifications and implications will rock the foundation on which the modern twentieth century was built. That word is **lifestyle**!

Our sedentary and relatively labor-free lifestyle has netted us more leisure time to do as we please. Yet we use more of our spare time than ever engaging in health-destroying habits. We eat more fat, eat more often at "fast-food" restaurants, and exercise more erratically than ever. Is it any wonder that a growing number of Americans are obese?

Our dependence on modern technology has unwittingly and irrevocably bound us to its advances. Each technological breakthrough allows us to spend less time on routine tasks of life that are now totally automated or achievable with the push of a button: the ease of a phone call, the faxing of a document, or the wondrously simple "point and click" on a computer screen. We do not need to expend as much energy getting our work done as our ancestors did. Life has become too "easy." Our physical bodies are not being physically challenged very much anymore. The one word that sums up our collective existence is: **sedentary**. Where do we go from here?

There may be a cure for the North American lifestyle that has led us down the royal road to obesity. This cure can be summed up in one all-important phrase:

Back to Basics. Many Americans have forgotten the best way to succeed in their endeavors: regular exercise, adequate rest, and eating a good selection of healthy foods. When it comes to a healthy lifestyle, we too often forget that it takes consistent and honest effort to achieve a desired goal.

Once viewed as a failure of will power, obesity is now seen by the medical establishment as a chronic disease. As such, it has stubbornly resisted a cure from all the best research that modern medicine has to offer. Its causes are varied and multi-factorial; its cure is as individual as the person it afflicts.

Many causes of obesity have been identified: biochemical, cultural, environmental, genetic, neurological, physiological, psychosocial, and more. The most common cause of obesity is the one that has resisted treatment more effectively than any other cause: overeating. Is it our weakness as a species to overeat? Are we genetically programmed to remain obese? Does environment play the biggest role? Or are we just bombarded with too many mixed messages of "Eat this" or "Taste that" while we worship thin models, swallow pills to curb our appetite and dream of our favorite high-calorie food?

It's time to wake up from our deep slumber of complacency and put our collective foot down.

Who needs to get up from that lazy-boy recliner and do something—anything? You do! Who needs to make healthier food choices and say good-bye to the empty calories of junk food that line the aisles of our supermarkets? You do! Who needs to teach children the importance of moderation and variety when it comes to eating? You do! Who needs to exercise? We all do!

In this book, *The End of Obesity*, you will learn about the basics of living a healthier way of life from two experts on this topic who are actively involved in teaching and refining their simple and healthy philosophy of living.

Introduction

As a family physician and author with a strong personal and professional interest in obesity and its management, I have long been aware of the common-sense philosophy: "You are what you eat!" My wife, Sophie Ares-Grief, RD, a registered dietitian who is currently pursuing a master's degree in clinical mental health counseling, shares my enthusiasm for a healthier lifestyle. She is blessed with a unique style of guiding her clients in achieving a healthy approach to eating through greater awareness of their daily food choices. Together, Sophie and I will take you on a fascinating journey throughout this book, reintroducing you to the simple and all-but-forgotten ways of approaching food and eating.

As you will realize after reading the opening chapters of *The End of Obesity*, talking about obesity is the most effective way for Sophie and me to help the large number of patients and clients that come to us for advice and treatment. Any problem has at least one solution, and the first step to take in finding a solution that is right for you is to talk about it!

Throughout the book, we have chosen to frame our comments as a dialogue between a family doctor and a registered dietitian. We have combined the latest information on health, nutrition, and obesity in order to present our views to you, our reader.

Our dialogue may seem a little oversimplified at times, but we do not apologize for this. Our goal is to present our ideas on how to end obesity in a simple, easy-to-understand fashion that leaves no room for mystery, doubt, or fantasy. Our ideas are not hocus pocus, nor are they revolutionary. They reach to the core of human nature and are truly basic. We feel that the simplicity inherent in our book's presentation will appeal to you as you choose a lifestyle that we believe in our hearts is the key to physical and emotional well-being and good health.

There is no step-by-step plan or guide offered here. You will not find the mentality of "jump through this hoop to get to the next obstacle" on the following pages. We will not chastise you or make you feel guilty for not blindly following the recommendations put forth in this book. There are many different possible paths at each stage of life, and we are here to help you find your own unique path at whatever your stage of life may be.

The goals you seek are universal: happiness, the freedom to choose, a life without hardship in the best possible health. Even though we offer suggestions throughout this book to help you cope with the difficult choices that you will face every day as you resolve to care for yourself, the emphasis is one hundred percent on you because you—and only you—can make good things happen for you. You can also make good things happen for those around you, but you can help others only after you have helped yourself.

We gently but repeatedly emphasize in our book the basics of how to eat well and feel good about yourself—at all times. New ways to approach weight loss seem to be coming not only from traditional medicine but from alternative schools of thought, too. In this book we do not focus on the alternative medicine approaches to weight loss. The forces of change cannot be stopped, but you can prepare yourself for change by learning and relearning basic, proven, and common sense ways to heal your body and fend off disease—and obesity.

The way to end obesity is by adopting your own set of rules that 1) makes you feel good, 2) does not jeopardize your health, and 3) you can follow without hesitation for the rest of your life.

We have chosen the topics in this book based on our combined professional experiences with our clients and patients. Here is a summary of the following chapters to help you prioritize your reading of this book.

INTRODUCTION

Chapter 1

Seven Steps to Losing Weight and Keeping it Off. Obesity is and has been a leading focus of most health-care providers and an obsession among the general population during the twentieth century. What better way to help bring an end to obesity than by using the word obesity itself as a way of promoting positive and healthy lifestyle changes? Dr. Sam redefines obesity as an acronym with his seven-step approach to taking charge of your own personal "battle of the bulge."

Chapter 2

A Dietitian's Perspective is our way of introducing the reader to the world of dietetics. Sophie outlines her own unique style of nutrition education in this chapter as it relates to an imaginary but typical patient. Dietitians are licensed professionals trained to offer the latest nutritional information on a wide variety of health matters. Each of us needs a dietitian. Have you seen your dietitian recently?

Chapter 3

In the chapter, **Time to Eat**, we challenge the notion that you must eat at set times throughout the day. The important lesson, "less is more," will result in positive change for you when you adopt the underlying concepts.

Chapter 4

Back to Basics: The Food Guide Pyramid is a chapter-long spirited interaction between Sophie and Dr. Sam emphasizing the underlying theme for this book. There are no tricks, no whistles, no bells for eating your way back into the shape you want. All it takes is a desire to return to the simpler way of approaching food. Go "Back to Basics" as Sophie and Dr. Sam enjoy a lively discussion in the comfort of their own kitchen, the food mecca of all homes!

Chapter 5

Sophie succinctly explains the importance of eating a certain percentage of your daily calories from North America's most dreaded food category, fat, in the chapter entitled **The Truth about Fats and Oils**. As you read about fats and oils, you soon come to a revelation: you need fat! We all do! Sophie helps dispel a few lingering myths about fats and oils.

Chapters 6-8: The Miracle Foods

With Chapter 6 we begin a three-chapter discussion of **"The Miracle Foods."** Chapter 6, **Eat Your Veggies**, will rekindle your desire to enjoy the abundance of healthful vegetables available from your garden or at the local supermarket.

In Chapter 7, **An Apple a Day**, we present to you a descriptive smorgasbord of fruits and vegetables that give you the nutrients you need for a healthy life.

By the time you complete the third chapter in this section, **Vitamins and Minerals,** Chapter 8, we believe you will be convinced that you need to eat a wider array of fruits and vegetables. Current research shows that fruits and vegetables contain high levels of vitamins, minerals, and phytochemicals (micronutrients that help prevent and reverse disease). In the light of new findings continually being announced to the general public, it is a wonder that Americans have been so slow to adopt these miracle foods in their diets.

Chapter 9

The emotional aspect of eating cannot be overlooked. We know that our stress-filled lives too often lead us to eat in response to our feelings and emotional needs. Sophie will explore the roots of this phenomenon, its

INTRODUCTION

impact on obesity, and new ways you can handle emotionally-induced eating in her chapter, **Mood for Food**.

Chapters 10-13

In the second half of our book, Sophie and I go on location to sites you visit often if you are a typical American. The goal here is to help you learn how you can eat properly any place at any time. Whether you are traveling, exercising, grocery shopping, eating out, taking a coffee break, or simply at home, making wise food choices is the basic foundation for a healthy body.

In the chapter entitled **At the Gym** (Chapter 10) we show you the best ways to incorporate good nutrition into your workout routine. In the next chapter, **At the Coffee Shop** (Chapter 11), we discuss the pros and cons of enjoying your favorite caffeinated beverage. Our chapter titled **At the Buffet** (Chapter 12) introduces you to the "out of ten rule," the visual appeal scale, and a new approach to beating the "buffet blues." The final chapter in this series, **At the Restaurant**, (Chapter 13) takes you to one of our favorite restaurants so that we can talk about North America's love affair with eating out. We all need to know how we would like restaurants to evolve as we prepare for a new century.

Chapter 14

The next chapter of our book deals with the future: our nation's children! **Children and Obesity** is a wake-up call to you as a parent, teacher or concerned member of our society to help our children learn the basics of good nutrition and better eating habits. Children deserve the best of everything, especially food. Starting the day off with good nutrition should be a child's "right," not a privilege. Children learn from adults—their role models. We need to show our children the right way to live and the right way to eat.

Chapter 15

"Magic" Pills is an up-to-date discussion of old and new treatments for obesity. The brief triumph of Dexfenfluramine (Redux), a short-lived pill in our war against obesity in the US, and more new drugs on the way, add to our confusion about the right approach to overcoming obesity. Will we ever learn that there is no magic pill that will put an end to obesity?

Chapter 16

"Wonder" Diets is our final chapter. In this chapter Sophie introduces her "hunger scale" as we talk about different ways people have tried over the years to lose weight. We leave you with solid information and helpful suggestions we know can help you reach your healthy weight range.

The search for answers to health-related issues, especially as they relate to nutrition and obesity, is the catalyst behind Dr. Sam's inquisitiveness and enthusiasm. Sophie's repertoire of nutritional information and her ability to convey easy-to-follow nutritional explanations to her clients are captured in our book's dialogue format. Ultimately, we trust that the respect shared between two professional health colleagues (who happen to share their personal lives, too) will help catch and maintain your interest and attention.

Respect your body and treat it well—and your body will reward you with a lifetime of good health. "The End of Obesity" can become a reality in our lifetime. Let's make it happen.

"Watch Your Diet?"

During my four exhilarating—and humbling—years of medical school, I learned more medical facts and medical trivia than you could imagine. All 150 plus students in my class were relentlessly bombarded

INTRODUCTION

with seemingly endless lists of anatomical, biochemical, and pharmaceutical facts—and that was just for starters. Add to that subjects like pathology, microbiology, histology, cellular biology, etc. and you begin to wonder how medical students survive this deluge of information.

As a student, the question that popped into my head almost every day was: Why do I need to learn this stuff? I'm glad I learned the answer to that question concerning nutrition, the one subject taught during my four fact-gathering years of medical school that, without a doubt, applies to all of my patients every day of every year of their lives.

Our medical school nutrition class took only one semester. Twice a week for twelve weeks we attended a 90-minute session on nutrition during our second year of medical school. That was all we were required to learn about nutrition. With this educational component we were considered competent in giving patients advice on every known nutritional problem, including high cholesterol, diabetes, and how to lose weight and keep it off!

One thing I was not taught in medical school nor during my two years of family medicine training at McGill University in Montreal was *when* to refer my out-patients for nutritional counseling to a nutrition professional—that is, a registered dietitian. As a medical student and a doctor in training, I did work closely with dietitians in the hospital setting, usually concerning patients suffering from diabetes, coronary artery disease, or other chronic diseases. This was great for my hospitalized patients, but what about the ninety-eight percent of my patients whom I took care of from my medical office? How could I be sure when to send my patient to see a "nutritionist"? Did I even know what a "nutritionist" could do for my patients?

It was not until I met Sophie, who later became my wife, that I finally understood the valuable role a registered dietitian could fill in the overall care of many of my patients. Through my conversations with her, I learned that nutrition is a daily event, not just something to think about once in a while.

Sophie has helped me guide my patients in learning the basics of proper nutrition. Even though nutrition is a science, physicians need to learn the art of communicating this science to their patients. Now that I know the principles of good nutrition, my patients can learn them, too. That makes me very happy!

If I could change one thing in the behavior of my fellow medical colleagues, it would be for them to stop using the following vague, useless, and paternalistic expression when giving dietary advice: "Watch your diet!"

In no way is watching your diet going to solve any of your nutritional problems, especially obesity. Watching something implies just that—watching. It is passive and involves not doing anything. Success in modifying your eating habits takes effort. You need to do things differently. Waiting around and watching is a guaranteed way not to achieve your desired goals.

So, stop watching your diet! The real way to reach your goals is to start taking charge of your health!

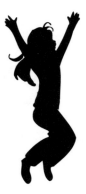

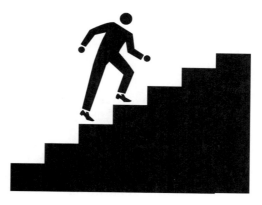

Chapter 1

Seven Steps to Losing Weight and Keeping it Off

"The only thing we have to fear is fear itself."
—Franklin D. Roosevelt, First Inaugural Address, 1933

WHY IS IT THAT SO MANY Americans have an overwhelming fear of being obese? This paralyzing fear prevents many people from losing weight even though they truly need to shed pounds because of health problems such as high blood pressure, diabetes, heart disease, or arthritis. Influential social factors help explain our society's obsession with obesity and our collective quest for thinness: the celebrity status of super thin models; exploiting potential miracle cures for obesity in the news media; magazine advertisements for weight-loss programs telling stories of people losing anywhere from fifty to three hundred pounds and becoming "better" people, and more.

There is no glory in our culture for those who are fleshly over-endowed unless you want to be a super heavyweight wrestler, a circus entertainer, or in the *Guiness Book of World Records!*

How can an obese individual conquer fear of obesity and be the healthy person waiting to emerge from within?

You only have to look your enemy in the eye and recognize that, to paraphrase President Franklin D. Roosevelt's famous line first uttered over sixty years ago, you have only one thing to fear: your reflection in the mirror.

For as long as the human being has been able to walk on two feet, men and women have been in pursuit of their daily source of sustenance and nourishment. When our earliest ancestors foraged for food with their bare hands and feet, even one meal a day was by no means a certainty. Human beings survived during this era of food insecurity by storing excess food (when it was available) as fat. In Chapter 5, "The Truth about Fats and Oils," we explain the significance of this evolutionary development. For now, we'll just say that fat is the most concentrated form of energy for the body. The ability to store food energy as fat has helped the human race to survive for thousands of years.

For most of the civilized and developed world today, life is not a question of whether or not a meal is available. Instead, we ask questions about how many, how often, how much, and what sort of meals we will eat in any one day. The abundance of food has given us the option of choice, but with all of those choices life becomes complicated.

We no longer view food as a means to stave off starvation as we would during a famine. We now consider food as a temptation. We say to ourselves, "Sure, I could eat an apple if I wanted, but I really would like to bite into that chocolate bar. It's daring me to eat it." "Sure, I could have a drink of water, but I really would like to taste the sweet, carbonated flavor of a soda pop."

For us, the idea of food no longer evokes fear over **whether or not** we will eat. Instead, food causes us to be fearful of **how much** we will eat. "Should I have three or six ounces of meat on my plate for dinner? One or two scoops of ice cream for a snack? More or less peanut butter on my bread? Eight or twelve ounces of juice in my glass?"

Quantity is our biggest food problem. The fear of eating too much food has led us down a path of despair. We over-worry and are guilt-laden about the big dessert we ate last night. To make up for our "gluttony," we deprive ourselves of the food our body craves (and needs) at the next meal. Later, we give in to our temptation for an extra bit of enjoyment and plunge face first into a luscious, heavenly piece of our favorite dessert.

Ah, paradise!

The result? Eventual weight gain. The effect on our minds? A conditioned fear of obesity. Pavlov, the late Russian best known for his Nobel prize-winning work conditioning dogs to salivate at the sound of a bell, would be amazed if he could see how so many of us have learned to fear our conditioned responses to food.

We urge you, whether or not you are obese, to seriously consider the seven steps in this chapter on how to lose weight and keep it off. These seven steps are offered in the hope that they will lead you to seek out and recover your own unique path towards good health.

Face it. Nothing in life holds more value to you than your health. Ask any person who suffers from physical illness what they would choose if they could have anything in the world, and the answer would invariably be "Good health!"

Good health is the foundation upon which you can build a happy and successful life. Most of us were born healthy. We grew up as exuberant, energetic, thriving children. As we became robust young adults we thought we had our whole life ahead of us. And we did, and still do, if we maintain our bodies in good condition.

As the body ages, a decline in physical and mental abilities is not inevitable. A well-oiled and regularly tuned automobile lasts a long time, and so will the human body. You cannot make a better investment than to keep your most personal and prized possession, your body, in the best possible working order.

By following a lifetime of preventive maintenance you will experience a higher daily energy level, a more alert mind, and a smoother and more efficient running "internal combustion engine" inside your body.

You want a "leaner and meaner" body? Here are seven thought-provoking steps to lead you on your way to a lifetime of energy and good health.

I have chosen to pattern my seven-step approach after the one word that is mentioned more often than any other medical word in this book: OBESITY.

Let's turn this nasty and ugly word into our best friend. We'll begin by making the word "obesity" into an acronym. "Obesity" is now a series of letters, with each letter representing an encouraging and motivating concept that you use every day.

OBESITY

O is for Overcome your fear of obesity.

You will not find it easy to overcome your fear of obesity because the problem is so tightly bound to our society's values. You cannot solve society's problems. However, you can begin to reach a personal solution when you recognize that the problem with you begins and must end with the way you see yourself.

Your harshest and most severe critic is you! When you look at your reflection in a mirror, what do you see? Do you see a person who is happy and satisfied deep down inside? Or do you see a superficial you—not enough attractive features and too many unappealing traits? Do you see the overall physical shape and form you have learned to accept, or do you see your hefty-looking hips, bulging belly, or over-endowed bottom?

I believe that within each of us lies the desire to do what is right for our body. We want to be physically appealing and in good health. We know we are more than just a mass of flesh weighing a certain number of pounds. We are thinking, loving, multifaceted individuals, whether or not we conform to the weight guidelines imposed upon us by medical research.

Learn to accept who you are, both inside and out. You will be happier and will be less preoccupied with your external physical self. If all of us would learn to feel good about ourselves, our society would not be so obsessed with external physical appearance. There would be much less pressure for unrealistic thinness that drives many women—and plenty of men, too—to shun any logical type of eating pattern.

Most of us fear obesity because of societal outcasting, social pressures, or medical ramifications. To beat down and overcome this societal fear of obesity, we need to reevaluate our sociocultural way of looking at food and meals.

o**B**esity

B is for **Bring your own meals.**

Think back to your childhood. Can you remember when mom or dad would lovingly pack you a meal for your school lunch and place it in a paper or plastic bag or in your favorite lunch box? One of my most memorable elementary school lunch boxes sported a painted-on picture of the cartoon character Fred Flintstone. My brother's lunch box had a picture of Barney Rubble.

Mom always packed me a sandwich: peanut butter and jelly on Mondays and Fridays, chopped egg on Tuesdays, cheese and lettuce on Wednesdays, and salmon or tuna fish on Thursdays—along with a fruit (usually a banana), a yogurt or canned fruit, a fruit drink (fruit punch was my favorite), and often a sweet dessert (my nickname was the "cookie monster"!). My mom always knew what I would be eating at school, and so did I.

Now that you're an adult, do you know what you are eating when you order out or go to a near-by diner or fast-food restaurant during your lunch hour? Unless you prepare your meal and bring it with you to school, work, or play, you are at the mercy of your favorite eating establishment.

You won't know whether mayonnaise, butter, salt, or anything else was added to the sandwich you ordered for lunch. You won't know if the meat or cheese in your meal was high or low in fat.

Does it matter? Yes, it does. When you bring your own meal, you know what you are eating. Knowledge about what goes into your body helps you gain control over your own health. Allowing others to prepare your meals for you is like stepping down from the position of captain of your own health care team.

Would you allow just anybody to organize your finances? And what about who you hire to take care of your children? I am sure that most or all of you would spare no expense or time to find the best candidate for the job. Would you trust just anybody to be in charge of your body? Of course not! So why trust a complete stranger every work day to fix your noon-time meal? Shouldn't you do it yourself?

A major obstacle preventing many of us from taking charge in the planning and preparing of our own meals is **time**.

Too little time. Does that sound familiar? Does your busy life prevent you from having enough free time to take five minutes to prepare your own meal?

The time you save not preparing your lunch in advance may tempt you to make more frequent visits to the restaurant. That leads to more calories because restaurants invariably provide you with more than you need to satisfy your hunger. By packing your own lunch you enhance your awareness of the foods you eat, making it easier for you to cut down on those extra calories.

To overcome your lack-of-time excuse, try preparing a week of lunch meals in advance. Or, try assembling left-over food after a weekday supper meal for the following day's lunch.

Pre-planned lunches give you a great way to use your leftovers. If you have any left-over chicken, for example, you can make chicken sandwiches, freeze them, then bring them to work as needed and keep them refrigerated until you are ready to eat. You can also save what is left over for a later-in-the-day snack, rather than going hungry and ending up munching on "junk food" brought in by fellow staffers.

Ideas for meals you can bring to work are limitless. Be creative, use your wild imagination, and go for it!

obEsity

E is for **Eat slowly.**

Have you ever thought about why restaurants such as McDonald's, Burger King, Arby's and others are called fast-food restaurants? It's not just because the food is ready to go before you've placed your order. People who eat at fast-food restaurants tend to eat faster, too. You should be aware that eating too rapidly can affect your dietary habits in at least three ways:

1. **Increase your food intake**
2. **Predispose you to indigestion more often**
3. **Decrease the pleasure of your overall eating experience.**

Of course, sometimes it is d ifficult to resist the tempting and aromatic appeal of food when you are hungry. Food tends to get shoveled into your mouth as your refined and discriminating palate is completely ignored. A good goal for all of us is never to let ourselves become ravenously hungry. If you are famished you are more likely to gobble down the food on your plate than if you are merely experiencing a relatively mild sensation of hunger.

As we discuss in the chapter entitled "Mood for Food" (Chapter 9), hunger is a combination of a state of mind and a physical-chemical reaction. From deep within the brain, a small area called the hypothalamus constantly sends hormonal messages to different parts of the body. One of the functions of this organ is to help us determine how hungry we really are. The chemical that plays the active role in setting and resetting our hunger level is *serotonin*.

When we eat, certain hormones and digestive proteins are immediately released into the circulation. These hormones and proteins work side by side in controlling how each food item is processed in the gut. As the stomach begins to expand and stretch with food contents, the message of this expansion is slowly transmitted to the brain via these digestive hormones. In the brain, a chemical message that the volume of food is increasing results in an increased serotonin level. It takes approximately twenty minutes for the level of serotonin to rise sufficiently in order to register "fullness" within the hypothalamus.

If you eat slowly, you will almost certainly eat less before your brain tells you it's time to stop. Don't be in a race to finish your meal. You may end up losing the race to your healthy weight instead of winning it.

OBE**S**ITY

S is for **Satisfy your cravings.**

Two widely held philosophies offer opposite guidance regarding what to do about your food cravings: fight them or accept them. If you fight them (as most dieters do), you quickly learn that you are fighting yourself.

Fighting your cravings creates a situation where you are depriving yourself of the food you want. When you finally give in to your cravings, the delayed gratification you experience often leads you to overindulge, resulting in a guilty feeling. You end up with low self-esteem as you berate and belittle yourself for not being stronger-willed. In the meantime, you resent the self-imposed dietary limitations. The end result: yo-yoing up and down the weight scale and feeling continued frustration and disappointment with your body image.

On the other hand, you can opt to *accept* your food cravings. You might think, "I'm in the mood for something sweet. I'll just have one piece of pie *a la mode*." You reason that the occasional indulgence is not a big deal. However, if giving in to your sweet tooth becomes a habit, this can lead to weight gain.

While it is only human to have cravings for pleasurable things, it is healthier to acknowledge your food cravings, know that you have them, and treat them as a part of your life, not as total enemies. Learning to accept your craving for a particular food item, and giving yourself permission to enjoy it may help reduce your cravings in the long run and reduce your overall feelings of deprivation.

Learn to appreciate all the flavors and textures of the food you crave to help you deal successfully with that craving. For example, one chocolate from the candy box can be succulently savored inside your mouth as it slowly melts on your tongue and on the inside of your lips. Using this method to satisfy your craving allows this piece of chocolate to act as a morale booster rather than taking on the added calories of ten pieces of chocolate—a real waist booster—to accomplish the same goal. (More on the above in the chapter "Mood for Food.")

You can also try to replace your food cravings with healthier food choices. Do you have a sweet tooth? Sprinkle a dash of brown sugar, a touch of honey, or a spoonful of yogurt on an apple. Make homemade applesauce with your favorite spices such as cinnamon and nutmeg. Indulge in a frozen fruit juice popsicle that you made in the freezer. Crave *healthy* sweets!

OBES**I**TY

I is for **Invent your own healthy meals**.

We all like to create new things. What better place to let your imagination loose than in everyone's favorite room—the kitchen!

For me, the kitchen has always been a place full of wonderful memories: watching mom bake chocolate chip cookies, eating mom's chocolate chip cookies, and inhaling those mouth-watering aromas that emanated from mom's home cooking! Only when I left my parents' suburban home and moved to downtown Montreal did I feel the need to learn the art of cooking. I taught myself to turn a random mess of food into an organized and tasty sandwich. Soon, I was tossing salads—and not all of it landed on the floor!—for family and friends. I experimented with baking, boiling, and steaming potatoes, noodles, and rice.

Preparing meals was a challenge I eventually figured out. I soon learned how to prepare an entire meal from scratch. Sometimes, though, I swallowed my male pride and asked my mother for a little advice on how to cook certain foods, like roast beef or chicken. I even learned a trick or two from my late grandfather, who at the time was living with me. He and I got along quite well, so long as we gave each other our separate work space in the kitchen!

To be honest, I spent most of my time away from the living quarters I shared with my grandfather for four years. During this time, I was deeply involved in medical school and my residency in family medicine. I was almost always too busy to cook, so Zaidie (my grandfather's nickname) would cook up one of his favorite meals for the two of us.

His recipes were simple—and fatty! We ate hot dogs, hamburgers, and fried potatoes covered in thick and creamy sauces three times a week. Zaidie had apparently never heard of cholesterol! Eventually I got tired of Zaidie's home-cooked meals and started eating out at restaurants on a regular basis. This eating pattern of mine led to a personal problem: my cholesterol level was 250!

Imagine the chagrin I felt upon receiving the news that my cholesterol was fifty points higher than the upper limit of normal. Me, a medical student, who supposedly knew more than the average Joe about healthy lifestyle. I was distraught!

When a bad thing happens it often ignites a person's passion to do something positive. I came to realize that my high cholesterol was actually a blessing in disguise. No more would I take my health for granted. No more would I be indiscriminate in my selection of food. No more of my *laissez faire* attitude and the feeling of invincibility that went along with studying medicine.

As I was agonizing over my cholesterol, a beautiful thing happened to me: I met my future wife. From Sophie I learned one of the most important health lessons I know: good nutrition can taste great! All you need is a dash of desire and a sprinkle of imagination to invent your own meals.

OBESI**T**Y

T is for **Talk about your weight.**

Talking about a problem, any problem, helps you focus your efforts on that particular problem. Sharing your concerns with someone who is interested but non-judgmental can help lift a huge weight off of your shoulders and improve your overall outlook on life.

Examples of problem sharing in groups include self-help groups like Overeaters Anonymous and Alcoholics Anonymous, as well as workshops on self-esteem or marital relationships, to name just a few. With any problem, talking about it and letting a trusted friend, a concerned group, or a trained counselor in on your dilemma does more than let you share misery with others. Turning to the support of others you trust can actually lead you to an answer to your problem.

Most obese Americans are able to share their thoughts and goals about achieving a desired weight. They struggle to exercise more and eat less, promising themselves that they will eat better and live healthier in the new year.

Sound familiar? You may fall into the above category. If so, do you find yourself regularly talking to someone about how you will lose your excess pounds and get back into good physical shape?

My advice: Keep up the fight! And keep talking! It is the heaviest and most severely obese individuals who have the hardest time sharing their obesity-related concerns with their friends, colleagues, and family members. Embarrassment is their biggest barrier.

If this describes you, I say: "Reach out to someone today and talk about your weight problem." Whether it is your best friend, your mother or father, your sister or brother, your spouse, your pastor or priest, a co-worker, or even your dog, there is likely to be a kind and caring pair of ears on the receiving end of the words you speak from your heart.

Perhaps I am a hopeless optimist, but I believe that a solution can be found for any problem presented. The secret is how to discover it. Talking about your weight is the first step down the path to your own unique solution. Problem solving usually requires a plan of action. What better way to make a plan that's right for you than by enlisting the help of a dedicated professional, such as a physician, a registered dietitian, or a mental health counselor.

Many of my patients tell me they appreciate the opportunity I give them to discuss with me openly their weight-related problems and concerns. And when I refer my patients to Sophie, my favorite registered dietitian, I know that they will find a caring person who will gently guide them through the tangled web of diets and the confusing maze of research studies in the expanding field of nutrition. I am confident that my patients will discover their own unique approach to losing weight.

Let's talk about obesity!

OBESIT**Y**

Y is for **You can do it!**

There is nothing better in life than to do something good for yourself or for the one you love. Telling yourself out loud that you can lose weight and keep it off can launch you on the road to successful weight reduction and future weight maintenance.

Every morning go to the mirror, look at yourself, and say out loud and with pride: "I can lose weight and keep it off!"

The most successful people in this world are not those who sit around while others toil. Truly successful people know that hard work, dedication, persistence, and motivation are the elements they need to achieve their goals. The drive to accomplish something good must come from within yourself. You must kindle a fire within your soul, your mind, and your heart in order to feel the passionate flame of desire to achieve your weight goal.

Success requires patience and perseverance. To lose weight and keep it off requires your effort each day. If you meet all of these requirements, the road to successful weight management will be smoother and fraught with less peril.

Short cuts are quick and easy but may carry huge risks. "Slow and steady" wins the weight loss race—every time!

How YOU can end obesity

O = Overcome your fear of obesity
B = Bring your own meals
E = Eat slowly
S = Satisfy your cravings
I = Invent your own healthy meals
T = Talk about your weight
Y = You can do it!

Chapter 2

A Dietitian's Perspective

"One should eat to live, not live to eat."
Benjamin Franklin

I AM GLAD TO SAY IT. I AM MARRIED. And not just to any lovely woman. My wife is amazing! She is a dynamic and self-assured person. Her words carry a wealth of information through her softly spoken dialogue. A registered dietitian completing her master's degree in counseling, she is the best teacher I know in the field of nutrition and proper eating habits. Allow me to introduce my partner in life and my extremely informed nutrition consultant: Sophie.

Sophie and I have collaborated on this book and will be discussing nutrition topics as they relate to obesity throughout the book.

This chapter is intended to allow Sophie to explain her approach in evaluating her clients' (and my patients') eating patterns as well as to demonstrate some of her methods in helping clients find answers to their nutrition concerns.

In this chapter, a patient of mine will be featured as an example of how Sophie and I work together in providing medical and nutrition counseling to our mutual patients. A few other patient stories will be included throughout the book, in order to illustrate the relevant health and nutrition points we are making. We have changed the patients' names and identifying details in their stories to preserve confidentiality. In the following story we have combined true experiences from several different people to make our intended point clear.

Joe Smith is a 48-year-old married man working as a senior accountant in a large tax firm. He was referred to me by a business colleague who is a patient of mine. In our initial conversation, Joe reveals what he claims is his *real* reason for wanting to consult with me: he is unable to keep up with his colleagues and friends when participating in business-related sporting events.

Joe's stamina for exercise has plummeted over the years, leaving Joe panting and puffing in front of his peers. This concerns and embarrasses Joe. Recently, due to his poor conditioning, Joe has begun declining invitations to outdoor sports events where he would have had to compete. "I look at the younger fellows of our firm as they throw the ball around and I dream about having their slim yet fit-looking bodies. I look like whipped cream compared to their firm cheddar cheese appearance! Doc, I feel I'm ready to start working on my weight, but I really need your help and guidance."

I ask Joe about his family life. He replies that all is well. He claims to be satisfied with his marriage of twenty-four years. His two children, a son age 20 and a daughter age 15, are both healthy and successful in their school and leisure endeavors. Joe's wife, Cynthia, is a successful florist who owns a floral shop in town. Joe tells me that his wife takes pride in her youthful appearance. In fact, she recently joined a group of her friends to form a mid-morning jogging club for women. Joe also speaks highly of his 20 year-old son (Tim) who is attending college out of state. These days, Joe only sees Tim on holidays or between semesters. On these occasions, mem-

A Dietitian's Perspective

ories surface as Joe recalls his own glory days as a college football player. As a student Joe took pride in his excellent health. He exercised four or five times a week at the school fitness center, kept his muscles taut and sinewy with muscle-targeted workouts, got his needed rest, ate sensibly, drank cautiously and, most importantly, had a positive attitude towards his general health and lifestyle.

After graduating with an accounting degree and embarking on his career, he met his future wife and began a new path in his life.

In the earlier years of Joe and Cynthia's marriage, they shared equally in the preparation of meals. Joe admitted to me that cooking with Cynthia had once been his favorite hobby. Recently, though, because of his hectic schedule at work, Joe has ceded his place in the household kitchen to his loving wife who now does all the cooking for both of them as well as for their children and guests. Joe admits he is less interested now in performing household chores than he was in his earlier years as a parent. Nor is it any surprise to hear that Joe is much less motivated now to exercise and work out than in those days of frequent five-mile runs and thirty-minute weight training sessions during his swinging bachelor years. "There just isn't any time for the things I used to do, what with all the meetings, deadlines, overtime, and paperwork at my work and home offices. Doc, I need more time in the day!"

Joe is in the midst of his own personal mid-life health crisis. He is representative of the many hardworking, decent, middle-aged people who struggle to provide for their families and themselves day in and day out. Joe claims that the sacrifices that he and his wife have made over the years were necessary to give the family all of the modern comforts of the late twentieth century. Nevertheless, Joe says he is ready to make changes.

The End of Obesity

I tell Joe it's time for him to give back to himself the blood, sweat, and tears he has expended over the years. I congratulate him for his new-found enthusiasm to tend to his most important possession—himself. Now he can run, bike, and pump his way back into the kind of man that he (and many men his age) would like to be: firm on the outside with well-lubricated joints, and free-flowing on the inside, both spiritually and physically.

I talk some more with Joe about his daily habits. He enjoys coffee and tea, but not to excess. Alcohol has become his way of relaxing. He drinks two or three vodka or gin martinis after work, and four or five beers on the weekend. Smoking has never been part of Joe's lifestyle. He learned his lesson about smoking years earlier when his father's oldest brother, Nathan, died at age 40 of lung cancer. At the time, Joe was just five years old. He would not have been aware of his uncle's death except for one unforgettable thing about Nathan: a strong aroma of tobacco. This powerful odor was on Nathan's breath, clothes, beard, hands, and especially in his car. Joe remembers the few times he went for a ride in uncle Nathan's Chevrolet. In winter, with the windows to the car shut tightly, the tobacco stench within the car would overwhelm young Joe, inducing waves of nausea and car sickness. Since then, Joe has never been the least bit interested in smoking a cigarette.

Joe's immediate family has not enjoyed the best of health. His father, John, died of a heart attack after two warning episodes of chest pain were ignored. John was only 50 years old. Joe's mother, Sarah, is 70. She has adult-onset diabetes and is taking medication for that. Joe tells me of a younger brother, Jim, who died in a freak accident. Jim was only 40 years old when he died.

Joe believes that his biggest detrimental habit of all is his love of snack foods. A day does not go by when Joe does not think about one or more of his favorite snacks—chocolate chip cookies, butterscotch ripple ice cream, or a nice, salty bag of potato chips. Joe has become accustomed to eating away from home. He frequents his favorite diner for breakfast, if he has breakfast at all, consuming the usual bacon and eggs with toast and jelly. Joe likes his morning coffee with one cream and two sugars. Joe's secretary often orders lunch: pizza, Chinese food, or a submarine sandwich. Joe usually eats supper in the evening at a restaurant with someone from work or with a client. Regular snacking on junk food such as chocolates, cake roll-ups, donuts, potato chips, and cookies, fills in Joe's eating routine for the rest of the day.

Let us now look at Joe's vital statistics:

Blood Pressure and pulse: within normal limits

Medication: none

Past medical history: nothing significant; generally healthy

The rest of Joe's physical exam and blood results do not reveal anything abnormal. Joe's height and weight are recorded: a height of 5 feet, 10 inches, and a weight of 230 pounds. Joe claims that his lowest adult weight was 180 pounds ten years ago and that his present weight is definitely his heaviest ever.

Joe is anxious to talk about his ideal weight. I explain to Joe that there is no longer such a thing as an ideal weight. Rather, we now talk about a healthy weight range determined by the Body Mass Index (BMI). BMI indicates your risk for developing weight-related diseases.

The BMI is designed for adults 20 to 65 years of age. BMI is not meant to be used for anyone with growth potential: babies, children, adolescents, or pregnant and nursing mothers. BMI is also not meant for the elderly population, endurance athletes, or very muscular people.

A person's BMI is calculated using height and weight measures according to the following formula:

First, convert height and weight measurements to the metric system. Jim is 5 feet, 10 inches or 70 inches tall. Since there are 39.3 inches per meter, his height is:

$$70 \div 39.3 = 1.78 \text{ meters}$$

and since there are 2.2 pounds per kilogram, his weight is:

$$230 \div 2.2 = 104.5 \text{ kg}$$

The formula for calculating the BMI (Body Mass Index) is:

BMI = weight in kg ÷ height in meters squared

$$\text{Joe's BMI} = 104.5 \div (1.78)(1.78)$$
$$= 104.5 \div 3.1$$
$$= \mathbf{32.97}$$

What does the number 32.97 mean? BMI is divided into four categories:

BMI 20-25 is a desirable range for most people. This category indicates a very low to low risk of developing weight-related diseases like that of heart disease, diabetes and high blood pressure.

BMI 25-30 indicates a low to moderate risk of developing weight-related diseases.

BMI 30-35 indicates a moderate to high risk of developing weight-related diseases.

BMI over 35 indicates a high to very high risk of developing weight-related diseases.

BMI less than 20 indicates underweight and may predispose to health problems such as anemia, heart irregularities, and others.

A Dietitian's Perspective

Joe's BMI of 32.97 places him in the category of BMI 30-35. I explain to Joe that his risk for developing weight-related diseases is moderate to high. Ideally his BMI should fall between 20 and 25 corresponding to a healthy weight range between 140 and 172 pounds. For Joe, we are realistically looking at the higher end of the weight range because he has a larger frame than average.

In summary, Joe Smith is a 48 year-old man with no previous health problems who is at the junction of two opposing and completely different avenues of life.

The first avenue is to continue to ignore his body's ever-changing situation and accept his progressive decline in physical endurance. Ultimately, Joe's lifestyle may lead to poor health and place him at an increased risk for many preventable diseases (see above). The end result: Joe's spending too much time at the doctor's office!

The second avenue is to buckle his belt, put on his exercise attire, and come on a journey filled with heart-pumping adventures, lessons in nutrition, and advice on how to prevent disease while strengthening his mind and body.

Joe decides to take charge of his own health. He is ready to make the effort required to do so. Joe says his objectives are to feel better about himself, live a long and healthy life, see his children marry, and enjoy his future grandchildren. The fact that Joe has come in to see me is a strong indicator that he is motivated to follow the second avenue of life. Joe is about to start all over again taking care of himself.

With encouragement, Joe is able to identify four goals which will help him attain his objectives:

1. Lose weight and reach his healthy weight range. Then maintain it.

2. Improve his muscle tone and strength.

3. Increase his physical conditioning so that he can be physically competitive with his colleagues.

4. Establish healthy eating habits.

To accomplish these reasonable and very important goals, I have enlisted the help of my wife, Sophie Ares-Grief, RD. With her comprehensive nutrition evaluation and her personal and therapeutic eating programs uniquely designed for each of her patients, we are able to direct more of my patients than ever before towards a healthier and more energetic way of life.

"Welcome, Sophie."

"Hi, Sam. Or do you prefer Dr. Grief?"

"Sam will do fine, thanks. Could you first explain to the reader what exactly is a registered dietitian?"

"Sure, Sam. A Registered Dietitian (RD) must have completed a bachelor's degree in nutritional sciences with an emphasis on food and nutrition, must have completed an approved internship, and must have passed a national examination. Registered dietitians uphold the principles and values of the largest nutrition organization in North America, the American Dietetic Association (ADA). The ADA's main goal is to teach healthy eating habits through promotion of the American Food Guide Pyramid and adherence to the Recommended Dietary Allowances (RDA) for all nutrients."

"There must be more to this philosophy than just following guidelines. So far, it seems pretty basic. Do you think our reader wants just the basics?"

"Sam, without the ADA's fundamental tenets, it would not have become the large and successful organization that it is. Its main purpose is to increase public awareness about basic nutrition and act as a role model for all Americans when it comes to making the right

A Dietitian's Perspective

food choices. Each member of the ADA upholds the above principles.

"Some dietitians have special training in different areas that may fit your particular health needs. There are some who focus on specific health problems, some who focus on athletic nutrition, and others who focus on pediatric, adolescent, adult, or elderly nutrition. Let's not forget those dietitians who specialize in vegetarianism. The list goes on and on. There are others, such as myself, who focus on the gamut of eating disorders, emotional eating, as well as obesity."

"Thanks Sophie. Getting back to Joe, I would love to hear how you initially evaluated Joe and what your conclusions were."

"There are thousands of ways by which registered dietitians go about teaching nutrition to their clients. As the reader will learn from this book, I have modified the basic formula for teaching nutrition in order to better serve my own clients. Now, I would like to give a detailed outline of the format of my nutrition consultation, and then proceed to demonstrate how it was applied to Mr. Joe Smith."

"OK, Sophie. You're on!"

"Even though there are many questions that I feel are necessary to ask my client during our initial one-hour session, most of the questions are fairly straightforward and require only brief answers. Occasionally, some of my clients' responses to my series of questions are anything but routine."

"You're saying you never know what is behind Door 1, Door 2, or Door 3! Let's make a deal!"

"Right, Sam. There is a structure to my interviews that I have formulated which helps me to elicit the maximum amount of nutrition-related information in as brief a time as possible. That way there is more time for my clients to talk about their underlying fears or concerns about food. Sam, you would be surprised how much people worry about certain foods. More about this later in Chapter 9, "Mood for Food." For now, let us look at a typical format for a nutrition consultation."

"Go ahead."

"It might be easier if I divide the entire consultation into easily understood parts, each with their own title and explanation. The first part is obvious. It is the **introduction.** During this part of the session I introduce myself, discuss the client's concerns and goals, and establish why the client thinks he or she was referred to me."

"Why do you ask your clients why they think they were referred to you? Isn't it obvious?"

"Not always, Sam. Often clients have been told by their primary health care provider that they need to seek the opinion of a professional dietitian. But many of the health care providers are vague as to why they are recommending a nutrition consultation. Their patient may have three different reasons for being referred my way, but to help my client the most that I can, it is extremely valuable to have them voice their own understanding as to why they came to see me. It gets the consultation off on the right foot."

"Do you ever see people who were referred by friends or family members?"

"Definitely. Some clients will even come in to see me without their physician's knowledge. However, as a general rule, I strongly recommend that people visit their doctor prior to the initial nutrition visit in order to rule out any other health problems. A doctor's visit may also entail blood tests and lab results which would also be important for me to know."

"I understand, Sophie. What next?"

"Part two of the nutrition consultation is called **data collection.** During this time, I go through my usual list of questions, asking the client all about current and past medical history, family history, current medications (noting any drug-nutrient interactions), vitamin, mineral or other nutrition supplementation, past diets, previous nutrition counseling, dental health, appetite changes, food likes and dislikes, food intolerances, food allergies, recent weight changes, and weight history.

"The client's lifestyle habits are also reviewed. Typical questions include the following: Who does the grocery shopping? Who prepares the meals at home? Do you eat out? How often? What is your level of physical activity? Alcohol consumption? and so on."

"Sounds like you pepper the patient with a whole slew of questions!"

"Not really, Sam. A lot of the data is collected even before we meet. A form filled out by my client prior to our interview covers many of the questions listed. I then go into more detail with my client as the need arises."

"Oh, I see. Please go on."

"I also take note of the client's height, frame size, and current weight. I calculate the client's body mass index in order to determine their risk of developing weight-related diseases."

"Great!"

"The so-called 'meat' of the nutrition consultation unfolds next. This part is called the **diet history and nutrition assessment.** A dietitian's technique in gathering details about the client's diet includes, but is not limited to, obtaining (1) a 24-hour food recall, (2) a food frequency questionnaire, and (3) food records.

"In a *24-hour food recall*, the client is asked to describe the food eaten during the previous 24 hours or on a "typical day." In my practice, clients are asked to describe their typical day's intake. I also acquire information on the preparation, cooking method, and portion size for each food item.

"A *food frequency questionnaire* nicely complements the 24-hour food recall or typical day's food intake. In order to get a cross-section of the kinds of foods that my client consumes, I ask how many times per day, per week, or per month the client eats or drinks various foods chosen from the different food groups. (See the chapter, "Back to Basics: The Food Guide Pyramid.") Even though the client may have eaten healthfully for the past two days in anticipation of the nutrition consultation visit, the food frequency questionnaire that I fill out with the client's help results in a more realistic picture of the client's typical diet. The answers to the food frequency questionnaire help round out the overall picture of a client's diet.

"*Food records* are another way of obtaining information about the client's current diet. This entails having the client keep a written record of his or her food intake for a distinct period of time, usually three to seven days. Doctors often request that their patients keep a food record or diary before visiting the dietitian. I find this method to be the least accurate because the process of writing down the foods eaten may be altered or modified by the client due to embarrassment about being truthful. Clients may also underestimate their food intake and omit noting certain foods, sensing that a certain food 'doesn't count!'

"Food records, though, do have their place once the dietitian has had a chance to explain their purpose and the specifics of how to keep these records. Following the initial visit, I ask my clients to keep a food diary of all of the foods eaten for two out of five weekdays and for one weekend day of a typical week as homework prior to their follow-up visit. The food diary helps my clients to remember the foods they've eaten. It is also a valuable tool in depicting healthy or unhealthy eating patterns. Most of my clients are glad to complete their food diary."

A Dietitian's Perspective

"Sophie, how do you go about sifting through all this nutrition information you've collected while the client is sitting in front of you and still manage to come up with a personalized nutritional analysis and plan? It sounds like it would take hours!"

"You're right Sam. The topic of nutrition is vast! The best way I know how to put together a nutrition plan that will work for each client is to 1) establish the client's most pressing health issue, be it obesity, hypertension, hyperlipidemia, or other, and 2) help the client come up with his or her primary nutrition goal, be it weight loss, lower blood pressure, a lower cholesterol level, improved eating habits, or other. With the nutrition information gathered throughout the interview, I am then able to offer specific recommendations according to the client's above needs and objectives.

"Sam, you may think that dietitians dictate what one can or cannot eat, but that is not necessarily so. Rather, a dietitian educates the client on proper eating habits based on diagnosis, shows the client ways to implement the recommended changes, and gives the client ideas on how to introduce new foods into the eating schedule.

"Just watch. Shortly, we'll see how all of the above applies to our hypothetical client, Joe Smith. Returning to my usual nutrition consultation, I end the interview by providing my client with a list of personalized dietary recommendations and specific ways to go about implementing the changes. This last part of the session is called the **wrap-up.** The wrap-up process helps to solidify all the new information provided to the client during the interview. During the wrap-up, we also have a discussion about the client's willingness and motivation to instill the dietary changes, as well as perceived difficulties in making such changes."

"It's important to remember that our eating habits are ingrained in us and reflect who we are as individuals. As a result, in many instances we are also referring to lifestyle changes rather than a simple food change. That's why handing out diets doesn't work."

"Sophie, I can see the benefit of using your counseling skills in helping your clients implement change."

"Yes, Sam. It's important to talk about the proposed changes with clients and how these changes can impact their lives as well as the people with whom they live."

"Do you offer your client any nutrition-related information to take home?"

"Nutrition handouts are fine, and they are useful in complementing the interview. However, a client will relate best to advice tailored specifically to his or her own personal needs. When I hand the client an individualized list of goals and objectives and ways to achieve them, the client possesses the essence of our interview."

"Excellent, Sophie. Do you offer anything else to your client before the consultation ends?"

"There are many great recipe cookbooks available in bookstores. Often, I recommend one or more of these cookbooks to my client. I also regularly give copies of recipes to my clients along with tips on food shopping, food preparation, and how to read labels in order to complement the important nutrition lessons that have just been discussed."

"Sounds like you cover all the bases, Sophie. Can you please share with us how you went about helping our mutual patient, Mr. Joe Smith?"

"With pleasure, Sam. The first time Joe came to see me, he was accompanied by his wife, Cynthia. I started off by introducing myself and explaining to Joe and his wife what the one-hour nutrition session

A Dietitian's Perspective

would involve so that they would know what to expect. I inquired about the reason for Joe's referral and what his goals and concerns were.

"At first, it seemed that Joe was reluctant to discuss his nutrition goals, although he later mentioned that he wanted to lose weight and improve his eating habits. During this first part of the interview, I sensed a noticeable tension between Joe and Cynthia. Using my training in counseling, I took a few moments to explore their marital relationship.

"I asked rather matter-of-factly how life was at home for both Joe and Cynthia. Cynthia was quick to respond for the two of them. She said: 'I don't understand why Joe comes home from work so late. He deprives himself of eating supper with his daughter and me and leaves himself so little time to exercise or simply unwind. No wonder he eats so poorly—he's always eating in restaurants or on the run.'

"Cynthia seemed to be harboring plenty of resentment towards her husband's busy work schedule and how it interfered with their family and personal life."

"How did Joe respond to Cynthia's concerns?"

"Joe said nothing. He was as quiet as a rock."

"Sophie, it seems to me that Joe and Cynthia were not getting along very well."

"Actually, it was only during Joe's follow-up session that he opened up to me and revealed important facts about himself. More on that later. Continuing with the interview, I proceeded with the data collection, inquiring about Joe's medical history, weight history, medication, exercise and other lifestyle habits. (See the details of "data collection" earlier in the chapter.)

"I then proceeded to the next part of the nutrition interview entitled "diet history and nutrition assessment."

"During this first session, I started the diet history by having Joe write down his usual meal pattern during

page 41

a typical work day. I sensed that in this particular situation, Joe would feel less intimidated by writing this information rather than talking about it. I then went on to do a food frequency checklist. The results were quite telling:

"Joe ate breakfast every morning at the local diner. His breakfast was usually simple fare, either bacon and eggs with toast and jam, waffles or pancakes with maple syrup, or cereal and milk. He would later consume yet another breakfast upon his arrival at the office, consisting usually of a jelly or glazed donut with coffee and cream. Joe never ate any fresh fruits for breakfast. He did not drink juice because he claimed it upset his stomach."

"Why did Joe eat two breakfasts? Was he that hungry?"

"Joe didn't say why at first. He just told me that someone from his office brought in muffins or donuts every morning. Temptation and habit led him to eat them."

"Okay, Sophie. What about his other meals?"

"Joe told me that his lunches generally consisted of either fast-food picked up by an office colleague or food ordered as take-out and delivered from a restaurant. Joe never got up from his desk at lunch time."

"I see."

"Joe frequently snacked in the afternoon. His snacks purchased from the vending machine at work usually consisted of donuts, mini cakes, and chocolate bars. When he finished work, usually somewhere between 5 and 7 pm, more often than not he would go out to a restaurant with a client or colleague, or drop in at his favorite bar for a couple of beers or a shot of whiskey before making his way home. As Joe put it: 'I'm generally not in a rush to go home.'

"Cynthia was looking away from Joe as he uttered these last few words. I thought I saw tears in her eyes."

A Dietitian's Perspective

"Sophie, what did you do next?"

"I asked Cynthia if she would like to share some of her thoughts. Instead, Cynthia grabbed for a tissue and said she would be fine. From that point on, I tried to continue with my nutrition evaluation. I asked if Joe usually had anything else to drink or eat later in the evening. Joe claimed he would often snack on munchies like potato chips and nachos later in the evening before going to bed.

"I summarized for Joe my overall opinion of his eating habits by explaining to him that his diet was low in fiber and complex carbohydrates (like bread, cereal, rice and pasta), deficient in bone-strengthening calcium due to a negligible consumption of calcium-rich foods, and sorely lacking in fruits and vegetables. Joe's food choices were also predominantly high in sugars, fats, and sodium. Given his family history of heart disease and cancer, his sedentary lifestyle, and his elevated BMI, I explained to Joe that he had a very high risk of developing cardiovascular disease, the No. 1 killer of North Americans.

"Near the end of our interview I again asked Joe the magic question: 'What is your most important nutrition goal?' His answer filled the air with hope like a ray of sunshine sheds light upon and warms a dark and dreary room after years of being sealed tight. Joe said: 'I just want to stop drinking booze.' Joe was now admitting that his alcohol consumption was a real problem."

"I'm not surprised, Sophie. So many people who suffer from the effects of alcohol have difficulty admitting their problem. During my initial consultation with Joe, he denied that there was any problem with the amount of alcohol he was drinking. I'm glad he felt comfortable enough with you to finally share his alcohol problem."

"From there I found out that Joe had been drinking to excess for nearly five years. His longtime relationship with alcohol became destructive following the death of his younger brother who died in a terrible car accident in which Joe was also involved. Joe told me how sad and upset he had been over the loss of his only brother and claimed he was still experiencing intense pangs of grief that alcohol helped to numb. Cynthia knew of Joe's longtime drinking, but didn't realize how many martinis with beer chasers he'd been drinking lately.

"As our interview came to a close Joe verbalized his desire to continue discussing the loss of his brother. I gave Joe and his wife the telephone numbers of both the local mental health counseling agency and Alcoholics Anonymous. Joe smiled as he got up to thank me. Cynthia's eyes were filled with hope. Then she got up and hugged me. Together, they left my office."

"Sophie, that was some nutrition consultation. I'm so proud of you. You need a big hug right about now, don't you?"

"Thanks, Sam."

"I know that Joe is doing better now. I saw him last week. What happened at his follow-up and subsequent sessions?"

"At his second visit, Joe came alone and was more verbal. As a result, he confided in me about many things."

"Such as?"

"Well, Sam, before I disclose to you what Joe shared with me, I'd like to remind you of the confidential nature of my conversation with Joe."

"Confidental, as always. Go ahead, Sophie."

"Joe had an affair with his secretary a few years back. The burden of not telling his wife of his infidelity was overwhelming. So he turned that much more to alcohol, his silent friend, to help drown his sorrow and guilt. I encouraged Joe to be more open and honest with himself. I asked him the following question: 'What do

A Dietitian's Perspective

you want most in life for yourself?' Joe replied: 'I want to be happily married and stay healthy.'

"Joe had taken his first step on the way to recapturing his health and his marriage. The rest of the consultation involved personalized nutrition advice. Joe learned about healthy snacking and alternative food choices for his sweet and salty cravings. I also taught Joe my simple hunger scale. (See the chapter: "Wonder Diets?") I reviewed with Joe the Food Guide Pyramid and encouraged him to learn to prepare his meals along with his wife. I took the remaining ten minutes of our session to teach Joe some relaxation techniques."

"I think I understand, Sophie. You're saying it's better to relax your mind and muscles with a do-it-yourself relaxation technique instead of drinking alcohol to forget your problems."

"Right. Joe's last session was very successful. Joe again came by himself. Our session focused on cooking and food preparation techniques, and on becoming supermarket savvy. We reviewed different ways of preparing low-fat foods. I also gave Joe instruction on how to read food labels. Joe said he was ready to go out and buy all the food for a great meal he planned to cook for his wife. A romantic dinner by candlelight, he said."

"Sounds like fun, Sophie."

"Lastly, Joe expressed interest in exercise. So, I referred him back to you, Sam, for further discussion on this and other issues of medical interest that Joe might have."

"Great, Sophie. As I said earlier, I recently had a nice talk with Joe in my office. He has lost fifteen pounds, has been 'clean and sober' for two months, and has started running and swimming after work at the local gym. He also wanted me to tell you two things. One, his dinner for two went off without a hitch. Two, he and Cynthia are going for counseling. They both feel that without your help, life might not be so full of hope."

"That's great, Sam. Joe is a true success story."

"You bet, Sophie. He even told me that he's eating his meals regularly at home and bringing his own snacks to work. He is looking forward to the next work-related sports-outing. He said he's ready for the challenge."

"Sam, how about a challenge of your own? I'll race you to the pool down the street. Last one in cooks dinner tonight."

"Sophie, you're on! I like my pasta *al dente*."

"Sure, Sam. So do I!"

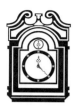

Chapter 3

Time to Eat

"No clock is more regular than the belly."
Rabelais

RIGHT NOW AS YOU READ THIS LINE it may be 7 am, 2 pm, 6 pm, or even midnight. No matter. Ask yourself this question: Are you hungry right now? Yes? No? Maybe? Perhaps you will look at your watch or at the clock on the wall and think: It is almost time to eat. Or is it?

Most of us depend on the passing of time throughout the day to help us accomplish our tasks and get things done. We set our alarm clocks at 6 am so that we can catch the morning bus or train. We carry agendas to tell us what, where, and when we will be doing our day-to-day activities.

Not surprisingly, during and in between all of this organized chaos that goes on in a typical day, we tell ourselves when we should eat. Let me repeat in case you were not paying attention just now: We tell ourselves when we should eat! Think about this for a moment.

Your moment is up. Are you still in a thinking mood? Good! As I mentioned, our busy lifestyles require that we schedule our time for work, rest, and play. We are all geared toward following the time of the day. It then should not be surprising if I tell you that even though you eat at certain times of the day, you may not always be truly hungry when you eat.

Sure, you tell yourself you're hungry and it's time to eat. But do you know how you really feel? Do you know the internal cues your body is telling you to indicate a real need for food?

Meals throughout the day need not be timed to the clock. That is, people should learn the concept of eating when they *need* to, not when they are *told* to.

During a normal work day, most people do not have the luxury of taking a "time-out" to eat when a hunger pang occurs. Most people have fixed work schedules that are not conducive to taking their snack break at a moment's notice. The average employee works eight hours a day with a lunch break of up to a full hour and two brief breaks during the work day. An executive or professional worker may put in ten or more hours a day and not take regular breaks.

Our society has imposed a one-hour "time out" near high noon (in the majority of North American offices) to allow us (force us?) to eat a meal. And we eat! The restaurant and food industry can attest to that fact. Americans love to eat out. The restaurant industry projects gross annual revenues in the billions of dollars every year.

Are you eating lunch at noon because it's time to eat? You may be wondering: What do I have against eating lunch? Isn't lunch an important meal to stave off the unbearable and inevitable urges for food later on in the day? Imagine modern life without lunch. What would we all do without our food break in the middle of our work day?

Let's see. Do we really need lunch at all? Let me put it to you another way: do we need any of our so-called breakfast, lunch, and supper or dinner meals at all?

What I'm saying is that our system of splitting up our daily food intake into three meals at fixed intervals (excluding our little snacks) is outdated, antiquated, ancient history, and frankly—all wrong!

Our modern society has led us down the path to food dependency from which we are all having a terrible time breaking free. We look forward to, anticipate impatiently, and even count down the minutes to our daily meals, especially lunch and supper.

I still believe in breakfast and am quite flexible in my definition of what constitutes a good breakfast. Originating from the root word *faestan*, an Old English term for not eating, the modern day "breaking the fast" has become known as breakfast. There is no traditional "must have" for the first meal after waking up from a night's sleep. There are an infinite number of ways to enjoy breakfast. Every person I know has a different routine regarding breakfast.

Why do I condemn our regimented and routine North American meal pattern but still accept, even encourage breakfast? Read on.

"Sophie, where are you?"

"What is it, Sam?"

"Do you have some time to talk to me about my favorite meal of the day?"

"Of course, Sam. Are you all worked up over breakfast again?"

"Come on, Sophie. Can I help it if I am so enthusiastic about the first and most important meal of my busy and fun-filled day? I would like to ask you a few questions and I'll give my two cents' worth as the need arises!"

"Wow! Two whole cents—"

"—Like pennies from heaven, Sophie."

"*Touché!* Sam."

"Before we talk about breakfast, let's talk about sleep and what happens when the body wakes up. The human body is simply amazing. As we sleep, our bodies go into a state of repose and repair. Whether it be for four, six or even ten hours, our bodies try to regenerate and prepare themselves for the coming day. Naturally, things are going on in slow motion inside our bodies while we sleep. Our internal motor is in low gear, revving gently throughout our slumber."

"Go on, Sam. This is interesting."

"Thanks. When we wake up from our 'beauty sleep' it's like a light bulb inside our body switches on. The body suddenly turns on most of its systems. These systems immediately begin to work, first a bit sluggishly, then with greater speed and ease. It's kind of like your car on a cold winter's day. Turn on the ignition and the car's engine comes to life. But try to switch into fifth gear too soon and you will be disappointed with your car's performance. The car needs to warm up and get ready for action.

"Same goes for the human body. As we 'warm up' after waking from our deep sleep, our bodies begin their daily tasks, all of which require large amounts of energy. This energy comes from our internal fuel. Of course, this internal fuel is the stored energy from our previously enjoyed meals. This stored energy, or energy reserve, is found in different forms in our body. One of these forms of stored energy found in our muscles is *glycogen*."

"Sam, can you explain to the reader what glycogen is all about?"

"Sure, Sophie. Glycogen is really just a big chain of simple sugars. Glycogen is broken down for immediate energy when no energy is available for use in the blood stream. Contrary to what some believe (and hope), fat, the body's premiere form of stored energy, is not the first to be broken down when there is an immediate demand for energy. It is only after most or all of the stored sugar energy in our muscles (mostly in our arms and legs) has been used up will the body begin burning its fat stores for energy.

"As we mention in Chapter 5, 'The Truth about Fats and Oils,' fat is a necessity for life. Fat provides more energy per unit weight than either protein or carbohydrate. Fat offers nine calories of energy per gram while protein and carbohydrate offer only four calories per gram. Perhaps you can now understand why people become overloaded with fat. The body is smart. It will store most of the extra calories we eat and drink as fat. This is an adaptive mechanism that has saved countless human lives during times of famine over the millennia.

"Returning to the human body as the car example, it is clear that without a fresh source of fuel first thing in the morning (or whenever you get up from your sleep) the body will not be able to excel at its primary function, namely: taking you to your desired destination and doing the things you need to do. Eating breakfast soon after you wake up for the day makes sense. Breakfast is fuel efficient and a must for top performance each day.

Breakfast Matters

"Let us suppose that our breakfast consists of a bowl of whole grain cereal with a glass of low-fat milk, a banana, and a glass of orange juice. As we eat our breakfast, our body immediately turns its attention to this new fuel. The food we eat is quickly broken down by stomach acids and propelled into our small intestines where most of our food's digestion takes place.

"Not surprisingly, the bulk of our food's vital components, including carbohydrates, proteins, fats, vitamins, and minerals, are absorbed through the walls of our small intestines. From there, our food is transported to various sites in our body for further processing and use. As the body utilizes the nutrients from our breakfast, it revs up its internal combustion engine, speeding up its overall rate of burning fuel. This rate of burning fuel is known to researchers, medical professionals, and everyone else as **metabolism**.

"Would you like to know the real reason I am a strong defender and promoter of the breakfast? Our body's metabolism speeds up to accommodate the fresh new source of energy we call breakfast. Following digestion of breakfast, our metabolism remains at a higher operating capacity. So, even though we have finished eating one hour ago, our body is still burning fuel. But now, it is burning our stored energy with greater gusto.

"It is important to understand this basic concept of breakfast as the most important meal of the day. Eating breakfast boosts our metabolism. So, breakfast has been, and always should be, the most important meal of the day."

"Sam, you really know how to push breakfast, don't you?"

"I still believe in the saying: eat breakfast like a king or a queen, lunch like a prince or a princess, and supper as if you were a pauper. Common sense demands that we adopt this kind of eating pattern."

"Good point, Sam. Why don't you elaborate on how the above eating pattern relates to our daily activities?"

"Sure. Most people expend the bulk of their energy between the hours of 9 am and 5 pm. Even though some of us work the late shift or have activities in the evening such as exercise, hobbies, social meetings, and more, our body's biorhythm cannot be denied. The natural biorhythm of the human body has crests and troughs, just like an ocean's waves.

"Our body's biorhythm is at its maximum between 11 am and 2 pm. To ride your biorhythm's wave and take full advantage of your maximum internal energy level during this time frame, you need to have the right kind and amount of fuel inside yourself to meet the challenges of the day."

"When is our biorhythm at its lowest?"

"Around 4 to 6 pm. That's why, near the end of a typical work day, it's natural to feel tired. To deal effectively with this normal feeling of fatigue, it's extremely important to choose what and how much food you eat during this low point. Too much food eaten at one sitting during this time of the day may result in feeling less energetic than if you had eaten a smaller meal.

"Eat too much at any one sitting and the excess is stored both as muscle energy (glycogen) and as fat. Sophie, I can no longer accept the status quo of big mid-day and evening meals as the only available options for our traditional meal choices during the 'main course' of our day. Allow me to introduce the concept of LESS IS MORE!

"That's right! Eat less food...more often. I strongly recommend this alternative approach to the traditional three square meals a day. This is where the concept of snacking comes into the picture. Frequent snacking throughout the day in conjunction with smaller meals is the preferred way of eating for weight management. The body is more efficient at burning calories derived from smaller meals and snacks than larger ones, thus leading to less fat being stored in the body."

"Sam, can you share with the reader the evolution of your message that LESS IS MORE?"

"Sure, Sophie. During my early days as a young and inexperienced doctor in training, a worldly and respected mentor of mine shared with me his simple views on how to be a successful medical practitioner. Of all the things I learned from him, this brief and paradoxical statement of advice stands out in my mind: LESS IS MORE. This concept has helped me over and over again in many different situations. For example, when I interview a patient, I know that the less I interrupt our opening conversation, the more I learn about what is troubling my patient. The less rambling I do in communicating with my patient, the less time the interview takes. The less time I spend on my high horse preaching, the more likely it is that my patient will actually listen to my words of encouragement and become a healthier person.

"We can now apply the lesson of these same three words to eating. Eat more than your body is able to burn off each day, and you will gain weight. What a lot of people do not realize is that just because a person is overweight due to overeating does not mean that this person's nutritional needs are being met. In other words, a person can be pound rich and nutritionally poor. What do you think, Sophie?"

"I completely agree with you, Sam. Often I help my clients learn the basics of proper nutrition first before confronting their weight-related issues. Overeating does not promise anyone a healthy and nutritionally-balanced diet. For example, think of a typical sedentary job such as truck driving. On the road for twelve to fourteen hours a day, the trucker stops for meals along the route in roadside diners or fast-food restaurants. The lack of fresh fruits and vegetables and the excess fat in a typical trucker's daily diet, along with lack of regular exercise, predisposes to obesity. This just reinforces the reality that for certain sedentary jobs and professions, incorporating healthy lifestyle practices into one's routine can be challenging."

"Before we go any further, can you think of any other ways to apply the concept of LESS IS MORE, Sophie?"

"Perhaps it refers to the type of foods we eat. That is, foods that are nutritionally dense."

"Nutritionally dense?"

"Yes, Sam. I like to refer to foods that provide a substantial amount of vitamins, minerals, and other nutrients with a small quantity of calories or energy as nutritionally dense."

"Quality not quantity! Is that where the term 'empty calories' comes from? Junk foods that provide you with energy but offer little or no nutritional value?"

"You got it, Sam. 'Empty calories' is the exact opposite of 'nutritonally dense.'"

"I truly believe that by eating smaller meals more often, with snacking in between, the American worker would be more productive, both on the job and at home.

"No more sleepiness after a big lunch. No more feelings of exhaustion after a large supper meal and dessert. Smaller meals, accompanied by frequent snacking, will lead to a pleasant feeling of satisfaction and an increased level of alertness accompanied by better overall productivity in those who choose to adopt this new and healthier way of eating."

"I couldn't have it better myself, Sam."

"Right, Sophie! All this talk about eating has got me hungry again, so I'm headed to the kitchen for a little energy boost. Want to join me?"

"I would love to, Sam. Afterwards, would you like to go for a long walk together?"

"You got it. Now, it's time to eat."

The End of Obesity

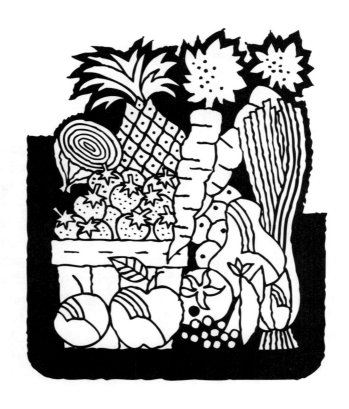

Chapter 4

Back to Basics: The Food Guide Pyramid

"Everything should be made as simple as possible, but not simpler."
Albert Einstein

"AM I HUNGRY! TIME TO RAID the refrigerator! Let's see now. There's leftover lasagna, fruit salad, muffins, Swiss cheese, cantaloupe. It's a toughie! Let's look in the freezer. I see leftover turkey, salmon loaf, tofu 'pups,' and my favorite sandwich bread: pita bread! What? No ice cream? I remember when I was a bachelor. Butterscotch ripple and rocky road ice cream were always in stiff competition. I never knew which one of these half-gallon ice cream containers I would polish off first when I was in my ice cream mood. And those chocolate fudge cookies I used to eat for dessert ...

"Thankfully, I've outgrown my unhealthy eating days and have learned to feed my body what it needs and not what the television commercials are telling me to eat."

"What was that I heard, Sam? Are you reminiscing about all that high-fat, super-sweet, melt-in-your-mouth ice cream you used to eat regularly?"

"Well, I—"

"—Sam, I have some free time right now, and I'm kind of hungry myself. Let's see what we can prepare for our meal by working together. What do you say?"

"Sure, Sophie."

"What do you feel like eating?"

"I kind of feel like eating something hot, but not spicy."

"That narrows it down a bit. There is the lasagna I made yesterday. Or you could have one of your favorites: melted Swiss cheese on pita bread with tomato sauce, onions, and veggies. Or you could heat up a soy-based "hot dog" or the leftover turkey from last week. Which one of these four choices strikes your fancy?"

"How about one of your famous Sophie sandwiches?"

"Sam, those are usually hot *and* cold!"

"That's right. Just like the baked Alaska I had at your friend's wedding. That was heavenly!"

"OK, Sam. You can come back to earth now. Need I remind you that this is exactly how you ended up with a cholesterol level over 200 and an even higher triglyceride level?"

"You're right Sophie. I should be happy that, with your advice, my cholesterol plummeted to 150 and my triglyceride level fell back to normal in only three months. That's one of the many things I love about you. You are level-headed and know what is nutritionally sound while surrounded by tempting and tantalizing foods."

"Thanks, Sam. But I'm only human, too. Now, let me show you how we can fix any number of tasty and mouth-watering dishes with what we have here in our very own home that you would want to eat every day, and twice on Sundays!"

"Great! I'm ready to learn. But please make it quick. I'm so hungry, I could eat everything in the refrigator!"

"Here, Sam. Munch on these sliced green peppers and cucumbers while I take out the food and display it on our kitchen island."

"Thanks, Sophie."

"Sam, before you and I whip up something tasty and nutritious, do you notice anything particular about how I arranged the food on our island?"

"Actually, yes. It seems like all the food has been separated into five small groups. Hey, I get it! The five food groups!"

"Good, Sam."

"But, Sophie. I thought there were four food groups."

"You're right. There were. In 1992 the United States Department of Agriculture (USDA), in conjunction with the United States Department of Health and Human Services (USDHHS), came up with the new idea of presenting the food guide in the form of a pyramid. This food pyramid concept has quickly caught on throughout North America. The diagram below of this Food Guide Pyramid is a graphic representation of all the food groups that were included in the Dietary Guidelines for Americans published by the USDA and the USDHHS.

"These updated and most recent dietary guidelines published in 1995 encourage Americans to 1) eat a variety of foods, 2) balance the food you eat with physical activity, 3) choose a diet with plenty of grain products, vegetables, and fruits, 4) choose a diet low in fat, saturated fat, and cholesterol, 5) choose a diet moderate in sugars, 6) choose a diet moderate in salt and sodium, and 7) if you drink alcoholic beverages, do so in moderation. The Food Guide Pyramid is a guide to daily food choices. This pyramid applies to every healthy person aged two years and older. The Food Guide Pyramid separates all the foods into five different food groups and advises us on the recommended servings per day for each food group. Let's look at the pyramid and see what it's all about:

Figure 1

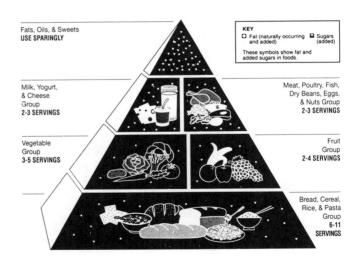

BACK TO BASICS: THE FOOD GUIDE PYRAMID

"As you can see, the base of the pyramid forms the foundation for a person's diet. This largest food group, the **grain group**, is probably the easiest for my clients and your patients to follow. Typical foods in this group include breads, cereals, pasta, rice, and bagels. An easy way to include fiber in your diet is to choose whole grain products such as bread and cereals made with whole wheat, barley, oats, rye or other whole grains. Choose enriched bread and cereals as these foods have certain vitamins and minerals added to them.

"Most people enjoy eating from this food group and therefore eat an adequate number of servings each day. A common problem arises when people start adding high-calorie toppings to their servings of bread and other foods found within the grain group."

"But what else can be used on bread? Toast is boring without a spread of some sort."

"This is where I help my clients learn to experiment and create new ways to enjoy their otherwise routine meals. As Francis Bacon once said, "Knowledge is power." Without creativity, knowledge is weak. Don't be shy to experiment. Why not try apple butter, apricot butter, or even prune butter as a spread in place of regular butter or margarine? Most of these 'butters' are just the fruit mixed with a bit of sugar and cider. Or why not try mixing low-fat ricotta cheese or cottage cheese with pineapple chunks and spread that on your bread?"

"Yum! They all sound like winners to me. Pass the apple butter, please."

"Not so fast, Sam. The next rung of the pyramid contains two food groups: the **vegetable and fruit groups**. Choose dark green and deep yellow/orange vegetables more often, as they contain a higher concentration of certain nutrients. Don't be shy to choose from a wide variety of fruits at your local supermarket. Be adventurous and try exotic fruits from time to time such as kiwis, papayas, and plantain.

"Five to nine servings per day are recommended from these two food groups combined. Sounds like a lot, doesn't it, Sam?"

"You took the words right out of my mouth. By the way, can you pass me a carrot stick?"

"Here, Sam."

"Thanks."

"These two food groups are on the same level of the pyramid because they are both considered of equal importance in one's overall daily menu plan. If you eat only veggies but no fruits, then you will miss out on a variety of vitamins and minerals. Eat all your fruits, but no veggies— same difference. Either way, you deprive your body of natural vitamins and minerals that help in a number of bodily functions needed everyday, including digesting and processing foods you have eaten throughout the day." (More on fruits and vegetables in the three-chapter section beginning with Chapter 6.)

"Sophie, you have just reminded me of a very touchy and extremely controversial topic: vitamin and mineral supplements."

"For as long as I can remember, I have seen television commercials, heard radio advertisements, and fingered my way through all kinds of health and non-health magazines featuring multi-page ads boasting of this or that vitamin pill's ability to boost you up and give you all the energy, nutrition, and proper balance of recommended dietary allowance of vitamins and minerals your body needs. Sam, have you ever seen in all of your medical readings over the years any scientific proof that these vitamin supplements improve a person's performance, increase their energy levels, or make them feel better?"

"No, I haven't."

"The American Dietetic Association's 1996 position statement clearly indicates that without empirically, random prospective scientific trials, there is no real evidence to support all these claims made in literally thousands of publications on a daily basis that vitamin supplements improve health."

"But what about RDAs?"

"RDAs (Recommended Dietary Allowances) are defined as the levels of intake of essential nutrients that are adequate to meet the known needs of practically all healthy persons. RDAs are recommendations, not requirements. Recommendations are made for healthy people. So, under the stress of an illness or malnutrition, a person may require a much higher intake of certain nutrients. RDAs are intended to be met through consumption of a variety of foods."

"Thanks, Sophie. Let's get back to the fruits and veggies. If I eat five potatoes and three apples a day, I'm all set, right?"

"Sam, variety is key. So is balance and moderation. Do you want to turn into a pumpkin? You will if that's the only vegetable you eat. Same thing goes for any of the fruits and vegetables."

"All this talk about fruits and veggies is making me thirsty."

"Here, Sam. Have a drink of skim milk. Speaking of milk, as we climb the food pyramid, the next stop is the **milk and dairy products group** along with the **meat and meat alternates group**.

"Yogurt, cheese, and milk make up the bulk of the milk group. Poultry, pork, beef, fish, eggs, legumes (dried peas, lentils, and beans), nuts, and tofu are examples of foods found in the meat and meat alternates group. Two to three servings per day of each of these two food groups is recommended.

"Unfortunately most adults, especially women, do not get an adequate amount of milk or milk products in their daily diet. That's too bad."

"I agree. Scientific studies show conclusively that bone mass is at its strongest in the 30-35 age range for women. Regardless of a woman's physical fitness or overall health, bone begins to "soften" after age 35, becoming less dense as the years pass. Many factors contribute to a quicker rate of loss of bone density. Yo-yo dieting or crash diets, for example, contribute to the problem because each time a person drops all that weight a bit of the body's calcium reserves are lost. If a parent, usually the mother, suffered from osteoporosis, there is an increased risk for the child to develop osteoporosis later on in life. Other factors leading to diminished bone density include not getting enough weight-bearing exercise, smoking, excess caffeine or alcohol consumption, certain medications, and of course, a diet poor in calcium-rich foods.

"The body is resourceful. If there is a low level of calcium in the blood, calcium is leeched from the bony skeleton of the body in order to provide an adequate amount of calcium where it is needed to sustain life. This is why it is important to provide our bodies with calcium-rich foods each and every day.

"Sophie, which foods can provide men and especially women with the bone-strengthening calcium their bodies need to stave off and keep at bay age-related bone thinning? By the way, don't mind me if I nibble on this cheese stick."

"For many Americans milk and other dairy products are the major contributors of dietary calcium because of their high calcium content.

"Milk is indeed the best source of calcium. The vitamin D in milk enhances the absorption of calcium into the blood.

"However, there are some people who will not or cannot drink milk or eat dairy products. Vegans (vegetarians who do not eat meat, eggs, and dairy products) as well as those who are lactose-intolerant and lack the enzyme needed to break down the sugars in milk and dairy products, can obtain dietary calcium through other sources such as broccoli, kale, turnip greens, Chinese cabbage and some other green vegetables, calcium-set tofu, certain legumes, canned fish, seeds, nuts, and certain fortified food products. By the way, when you enjoy canned fish, don't forget to mash up the bones and eat them, too. Calcium-fortified juices are now also available."

"Great! What about the meat and meat alternates group, Sophie?"

"This is a real problem for most North Americans. As you know, the majority of Americans are meat eaters. I don't believe that this in itself is necessarily a bad thing, although there are those who might disagree. I believe the problem with our collective North American diet is that meat has become the center of our attention.

"Look at the menu of any non-vegetarian restaurant in North America. My guess is that over 95 percent of these restaurants have as their star attraction a meat or other protein source such as poultry or fish. Whether it is red meat, chicken, turkey, lamb, ham, veal, or any other type of protein, the question that we never fail to think if not ask is, 'Where's the meat?'"

"Sophie, what's wrong with having a piece of meat for supper? Right now, I have a terribly strong craving for a roast beef sandwich with all the trimmings!"

"Actually, from a nutrition standpoint, there is nothing wrong with eating two to four ounces of lean meat for supper, lunch, or even breakfast. The problem arises when portion sizes are larger than what the body requires. Restaurants are notorious for serving their customers a big portion of meat.

"For those of us blessed with good health, including a well-conditioned heart, well-aerated lungs, and efficiently functioning kidneys, we can usually process and metabolize meat relatively quickly without incident. However, ask an already overworked heart, poorly ventilated lungs, and inefficient kidneys to break down, filter, and eliminate an excess amount of protein and you are asking for trouble.

"Our kidneys are the body's premiere organs with respect to filtration. Almost every food you eat and beverage you drink is filtered through your kidneys. The body needs a certain amount of protein to function at peak efficiency. However, once your body has obtained that amount of protein, the kidneys are left with the heroic challenge of filtering the remaining protein in the blood. You see, the body cannot store its excess protein like it does excess fat. Protein needs to be eliminated.

"Filtering protein is hard work for the kidneys. If your kidneys are asked over and over to filter an excess amount of protein, the result can be worn-out kidneys— a serious problem!

"Another problem with eating too much meat is the excess fat that often hides within the meat—especially red meat. As the reader probably knows, excess fat in the diet is a major culprit in the two leading causes of death in North America: heart attack and stroke. It is a sad fact that so many of these deaths are preventable. One way of reducing this twentieth century epidemic of cardiovascular disease is to learn to eat less meat and to eat healthier and leaner cuts of meat."

"Sophie, I agree with you that certain meats are fattier than others. I also know that too much of a good thing can become a bad thing. But can't a guy or a gal enjoy a nice, juicy piece of steak, cooked on the grill to perfection, with a bit of seasoning and sauce, and not feel guilty about it every time?"

"Of course, anyone can enjoy their steak and eat it, too! The point is that Americans are doing that all the time. Millions of people eat meat to excess on a daily basis and their bodies are regretting it. Moderation, as always, is the key to a healthy and energetic existence. That is the message here."

"Sophie, I totally agree with moderation. So, what can I eat instead of my steak?"

"Sam, you don't have to avoid steak entirely. We can still have our summer barbecues and go out to your favorite steak house now and then. The point of this discussion is to encourage the reader to eat less meat...less often.

"When the average American family sits down at the dinner table tonight, I hope that instead of serving themselves a big piece of meat, they will serve less meat, enjoy it more, and complement their meat with a variety of foods from the other food groups.

"I challenge the reader to come up with any variation of non-meat side dishes that can be used interchangeably and regularly. We would all be healthier and suffer less disease if meat were to become the side dish in all of our meals."

"Interesting concept, Sophie. Are we now ready to prepare our meals?"

"Just one more group, Sam. This group is the one that everyone focuses their attention on even though we need only a small amount of it to keep us going. I am talking about the **Fats and Oils** food group."

"Sophie, let's leave the fats and oils for next chapter. I'm ready to get cooking!"

"All right, Sam. Let's get busy!"

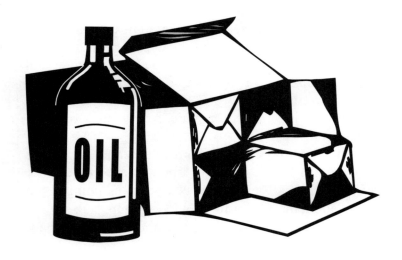

Chapter 5

The Truth about Fats and Oils

"The pure and simple truth is rarely pure and never simple."
Oscar Wilde

THE TRUTH IS THAT IF WE didn't have fat we would die! It is shocking that such a small word can represent something so important to life. What's even more bewildering is our continuous and seemingly endless struggle as a species to get rid of fat.

Love it or hate it, fat is a part of our bodies. We need fat. Without it, we would not have any protective insulation. Our bodies would be poorly suited to fend off the coldest winter day, even with clothing. Without fat, we would have less cushion to protect our bones from the daily bumps and bruises of modern living.

Like all nutrients, fat is beneficial and required in appropriate quantities. Fat is the vehicle through which we obtain several life-sustaining vitamins such as vitamins A, D, E, and K. These fat-soluble vitamins are crucial to the normal functioning of our bodies.

Fat also serves in the making of certain hormones and is responsible for maintaining the structure and health of, as the late astronomer Carl Sagan might have said, "the billions and billions of cells in the body."

The fact is that the human body will convert excess food eaten at any one meal into our society's most maligned and talked about energy system: **FAT**. Our body stores excess food energy as fat because, in times of famine, fat provides more energy per unit weight than any other form of stored energy available for internal human combustion.

Face it, your body likes having *some* fat. Ideally, American adults should consume no more than 30 percent of their day's total energy intake from fat. The sad reality is that Americans derive anywhere from 35 to 40 percent of their total calories from fat.

In the past, industries incorporated fats and oils into foods in order to give these foods more palatability, flavor, aroma, and tenderness. Over the years, the practice of imparting foods with a fatty, oily feeling has all but disappeared. Food manufacturers have sensitized themselves to the needs and wants of the consumer. They have re-engineered many of their ingredients so that their food products can be labeled as "low-fat" or "fat-free."

Since more and more Americans are buying these lower-fat and non-fat versions of foods, why is it that so many Americans are still obese? Despite all the fat-free products on the market, Americans are still not achieving a deficit in calories. *Americans have not significantly reduced their total calorie intake and are still not exercising sufficiently.*

Don't be fooled! Just because a food is labeled as fat-free does not mean it is calorie-free! Many products that are fat-free contain extra sugar to enhance their taste. It should be no surprise that some of the fat-free products in your local grocery store actually *contain more calories* than their fat-containing counterparts!

When reducing or modifying your fat consumption, it is important to be familiar with the different types of fats found in our diet. All fats contain a proportion of saturated, monounsaturated and polyunsaturated fats.

Saturated fats are found mainly in or derived from animal sources. Fatty meats, butter, cream, ice cream, high-fat milk and high-fat dairy products are all examples of foods rich in saturated fats. Please be aware that saturated fats have a powerful cholesterol-raising effect.

Although coconut oil (92 percent saturated), palm kernel oil (82 percent) and palm oil (51 percent) are vegetable oils not derived from animal sources, they are naturally high in saturated fats. These vegetable oils are often used in commercial baked goods like cakes, pies, cookies and are known as "hidden fats."

Another type of hidden fat is **hydrogenated** fat. Vegetable oils are hydrogenated (hardened) by a chemical procedure called hydrogenation. Hydrogenation is used in the production of some margarine and many baked goods and candies. This process involves adding hydrogen to a liquid oil, thus making it easier to spread this "hardened oil" at room temperature. Hydrogenation also enhances the shelf life of the food. The main reason hydrogenation has been scrutinized of late is terribly simple: in the body, hydrogenated fat behaves as a harmful saturated fat!

The next category of fat is the **monounsaturated** fats. These fats are derived from vegetable sources and are liquid at room temperataure. Examples of oils with a high mono-unsaturated fat content include olive oil (77 percent mono-unsaturated), canola oil (58 percent) and peanut oil (48 percent).

Examples of foods with a high mono-unsaturated fat content include olives, avocados, nuts, and seeds.

Studies have shown that monunsaturated fats do not have any effect on increasing or lowering the blood cholesterol. Further studies have also indicated that replacing saturated fats with monounsaturated fats in our diet can help reduce the bad cholesterol known as LDL. LDL (Low Density Lipoprotein) is actually a protein which binds to the blood cholesterol and deposits the cholesterol onto the lining of arteries. Monounsaturated fats do not have any effect on a person's HDL (High Density Lipoprotein). HDL, known as the good cholesterol, removes the cholesterol from the arteries and delivers it to the liver for elimination from the body. (See Chapter 10, "At the Gym," for more details on LDL and HDL.)

The last category of fat is **polyunsaturated** fats. These fats are also derived from vegetable sources and are liquid at room temperature. Examples of oils rich in polyunsaturated fats include safflower oil (78 percent polyunsaturated), sunflower oil (69 percent), corn oil (62 percent), and soybean oil (61 percent).

Replacing saturated fats with polyunsaturated fats can also help reduce bad cholesterol levels (LDL). However, studies have shown that too much of the polyunsaturated fats in our diet can also reduce a person's HDL level.

The take-home message here is this: It is a good idea to be careful of how much fat goes into your diet. However, it would not be a good idea to eliminate all fats from your diet. Choose heart-healthy fats such as monounsaturated and polyunsaturated fats more often than saturated fats and use all of them in reasonable amounts. Remember, **variety** and **moderation** are the keys to your success.

What about Olestra, the new fat replacer?

Olestra (brand name "Olean") is a "fat-free" fat developed by the Procter and Gamble Company. It is referred to as fat-free because it passes through the gastrointestinal tract without being digested or absorbed. Olestra was granted FDA (Food and Drug Administration) limited approval in the United States for use in crackers and non-sweet snacks such as cheese puffs, potato chips, tortillas, and corn chips. Olestra tastes like "real" fat and can be used in baking and frying without contributing a single calorie.

Olestra has been said to be non-toxic. However, it does have certain negative physiological effects. Two are mentioned here. The first one is a reduced absorption of fat-soluble nutrients, particularly carotenoids and vitamins A, D, E, and K. These nutrients attach themselves to Olestra and pass directly through the body without being absorbed. It's as if these nutrients were never there! The second one has greater potential for social unacceptability: Olestra can also provoke *anal leakage* and even diarrhea because of its liquid thin consistency.

The manufacturer has addressed the above concerns by adding supplemental vitamins A, D, E, and K to foods containing Olestra, and by making Olestra more viscous in order to slow down its passage through the gut and lessen the risk of diarrhea.

Procter & Gamble has not attempted to compensate for the loss of carotenoids because their health benefits, such as safeguarding against certain types of cancer, heart disease, and macular degeneration (diminished eyesight in the elderly) have not yet been scientifically proven. Some argue that carotenoid depletion occurs only when Olestra and carotenoids are eaten at the same time.

The question is whether Olestra will reduce the fat and consequently the total calorie intake of America's diet. This won't happen if people who eat products containing Olestra make up for their savings in calories by eating too much fat-free and other calorie-reduced foods. Remember, fat-free does not mean calorie-free. If you eat snack foods made with Olestra, do so in moderation.

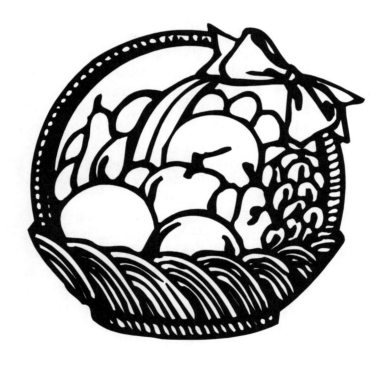

The Miracle Foods

An Introduction to Chapters 6, 7, 8

"Man must go back to nature for information."
Thomas Paine

BIOLOGY. REMEMBER THAT WORD. Chemistry. Don't forget that word, either. Marry the two words and you get **biochemistry**.

The living human being (that's us) is an amazing biochemical phenomenon. Millions of intricate reactions occur flawlessly every hour within our bodies to keep them orderly and running smoothly. We all depend on this biochemical network of events inside every cell of our bodies. It takes only one mutation of one little piece of one of literally trillions of building blocks in our complex body to create havoc in our design. Think of it: only one mistake in trillions of sophisticated biochemical equations is all it takes for the body to falter and possibly break down. Incredible!

This section of our book is about the foods we need to embrace with a passion. These foods are the product of millions of years of natural evolution and are fit for us to eat. They are survivors from the past that are now beckoning us to come and get them. These wondrous, life-saving foods are our biochemical saviors. Without further ado, we introduce you to the miracle foods: **fruits and vegetables.**

Once used as medicines, fruits and vegetables have long since lost their position among the ranks of nature's wonders. With our recent technological advances and improved capabilities to study and analyze the foods we eat, some startling evidence has surfaced. Study after study overwhelmingly link the consumption of fruits and vegetables with a lower likelihood of developing a myriad of diseases. Evidence is mounting that eating fruits and vegetables lowers the risk of cancer of the mouth, pharynx, esophagus, stomach, pancreas, colon, lung and endometrium. Other diseases that occur much less frequently among people who eat more of nature's miracle foods include cardiovascular disease, diabetes, stroke, diverticulosis, and the disease that is the focus of this book: **OBESITY.**

How do these miracle foods work their wonders? Simple. It's biochemistry! After years of investigating fruits and vegetables, researchers have discovered biochemical compounds within these foods that have a major effect on our biological selves. These biochemical substances hold the secret to much of what ails us. Many of these cancer-reducing and disease-preventing substances can be found only in fruits and vegetables.

Most of these life-saving biochemical rescuers are known as **vitamins** and **minerals**. Others that are more obscure but becoming better known include *allium compounds*, found in onions, garlic, scallions, leeks, and chives; *carotenoids*, found in fruits and vegetables with an orange or yellow color; *dithiolthiones*, found in cruciferous vegetables such as cabbage, brussels sprouts, cauliflower and broccoli; *isoflavones*, found in soybeans, and many more. Although not technically biochemical, the **fiber** content of fruits and vegetables

The Miracle Foods—An Introduction

is noteworthy and abundant. Fiber helps protect us from potentially toxic digestive by-products of the foods we eat by increasing the speed at which these potentially poisonous substances and metabolic wastes pass out of our bodies.

When all the evidence is in (and scientific proof accumulates on a daily basis), the verdict will be clear and compelling: fruits and vegetables are our biochemical friends. Their safety net is large and inviting. All we have to do is jump in.

Collectively, let's raise the average intake of fruits and vegetables in the US from the low current rate of 3.4 servings per day to between 5 and 9 servings per day. We will all be better off, as individuals and as a society.

The most important nutritional advice you will ever get from your physician or other health care provider is this: "Eat five or more fruits and vegetables a day." When you hear this, listen! It can lead you down the road to better health.

Now come with us as we learn more about nature's wonderful gifts: fruits and vegetables, and their vitamins and minerals.

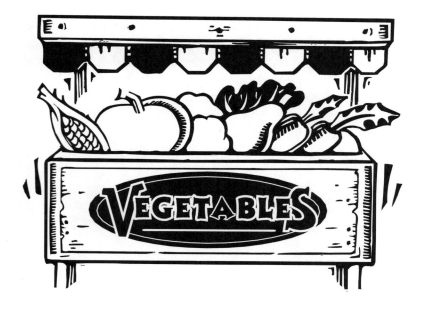

The Miracle Foods, Part 1

Chapter 6

Eat Your Veggies!

"I like my spinach."
Popeye

A CONCERNED AND LOVING PARENT can experience no greater thrill than to see a son or daughter blossom into a healthy and vibrant teenager. However, before the pubescent transformation occurs, a child has to learn much about life—mostly from the parents.

Among other things, a child should be taught proper eating habits and appropriate attitudes towards food at the family dinner table. When I was a boy, my parents subscribed to the belief that not finishing every morsel of food on your dinner plate was a serious offense that merited a memorable punishment—no TV for me! As a result, I can count on only one hand the number of times during my childhood when I did not finish my supper. Television was that important to me!

This universally shared parental hope that all children will grow up healthy and happy is often supplemented by well-known phrases that parents are notorious for using at the dinner table. A common and overused exhortation of my parents was, "Eat your veggies!"

During my childhood years, all vegetables looked and tasted the same to me—blah! Eventually, I learned to like mom's mashed potatoes. It took me ten years before I was able to fully appreciate the entire range of mom's cooking, especially her vegetable dishes.

As soon as I developed a taste for veggies, there was no stopping me. I would eat any vegetable, no matter what color or size. I even learned to like the one vegetable that had eluded my taste buds for years: brussels sprouts!

Another vegetable also had to fight its way onto my plate: yellow corn. Every year around the end of summer, my father would drive our family from Montreal to Long Island, New York, to visit our American relatives. Each visit there brought us into contact with the best mixed yellow and white corn on the cob I had ever tasted! From then on, I refused to eat plain yellow corn! I wanted yellow and white corn. It took another decade for me to regain some desire for yellow corn. To this day, whenever I eat corn on the cob, I fondly remember those lazy summer days during my childhood when I tasted the golden and cream-colored niblets of country fresh corn.

My childhood experiences with vegetables are certainly not uncommon. Children generally shy away from foods that are not naturally sweet as they begin to experiment with the novel and powerful tastes and smells of new foods. It is a fact that all of us, including children, have taste buds that naturally steer us toward eating sweet and salty foods. All other foods are an acquired taste.

For children, learning to savor the textures and flavors of foods can be made easier if their parents introduce a new food in a fun and interesting manner. This applies especially to the one food group that all kids seem born to dislike: vegetables. Getting a child to eat veggies may be very challenging for parents. The biggest reasons why children don't like vegetables can be summed up in three phrases:

> 1) **vegetables are not fun**
>
> 2) **vegetables taste strange to a child's immature palate**
>
> 3) **vegetables look weird!**

For example, why don't children like asparagus? Did you like asparagus at age six? Could you even pronounce it then? Vegetables are just too foreign for our kids. They cannot understand why they need their veggies.

Telling boys that eating spinach will "grow hair on your chest" or telling girls that "eating broccoli will give you beautiful hair" doesn't work now and never did. The trick to getting your child interested in vegetables is to make buying, preparing, and eating them an exciting event.

Instead of boiled spinach and boring broccoli on the plate, how about "carrot hockey sticks," "green pepper baseball bats," "broccoli bouquets," or "green pea necklaces"? Use your imagination to transform veggies into cute little objects that are fun to eat.

Vegetables are not just for vegetarians. We all should eat an eclectic mix of these nutrient-rich foods on a daily basis. Vegetables are unbelievably full of nutrition. Some provide a whole day's supply of certain important vitamins and minerals. With a little imagination and creativity, we can make vegetables as interesting and enjoyable to eat as a nice, juicy piece of filet mignon steak is to meat eaters.

The overwhelming variety of vegetables available in our supermarkets and grocery stores is a testament to how important vegetables are to our society and the rest of the world.

Vegetables deserve to be at the top of our shopping list. And they should be on our plates every night. Whether you boil, microwave, oven cook, dice, chop, slice, or mash your veggies, there is something I want you to remember: The best way to profit from all of the natural benefits of these miracle foods is to **eat your veggies**!

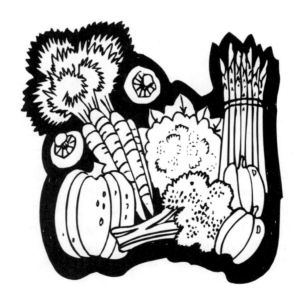

The Miracle Foods, Part 2

Chapter 7

An Apple a Day

"Variety is the spice of life."
Cowper, The Task, II

IT IS SAFE TO SAY THAT MOST PEOPLE in North America and around the world know what a fruit is: an edible product that grows from a plant or tree.

How important are fruits to us, anyway? You only have to look in your local supermarket or grocery store's produce section to see the bountiful variety of colorful fruits piled up high for your appreciation and selection to get an idea of how much value our society places on fruits.

Fruits are great food items. Most fruits can be eaten as is, without any special preparation. Fruits are chock full of vitamins and minerals, have virtually no fat, and are a good source of energy for the active person.

Yet few North Americans eat the USDA recommended minimum quantity of two to four servings of fruit per day. Why is that? Are fruits hard to come by? Hardly. Their overabundance is impossible to notice. Do fruits taste bad? I don't think so, unless you have the misfortune of having no taste buds. Are fruits too expensive for people to buy? No more so than cakes and cookies.

In reality, we often eat "fruity alternatives" instead of real fruit. Fruit pops, fruit cakes, fruit-flavored sodas, and other products with a link to a fruit are plentiful in our stores and homes. An entire industry based solely on fruit juices and fruit drinks has existed for over a quarter of a century. Orange juice, lemonade, apple cider, and of course, wine are excellent examples of products derived directly from fruits that we have come to love and appreciate.

Our strong interest in drinking juice has spawned all kinds of mechanical and electrical "juicers" to extract nutritional value from fruit. I believe that nature intended for us to eat fruits as they are and with our teeth.

Biting into and chewing a piece of fresh fruit is an experience to be savored. This natural way of eating fruits should not be replaced by sipping fruit juice from a straw. By drinking our fruit we miss out on a very important ingredient for good health: FIBER!

Dietary fiber is plant material that is eaten but not digested. Fiber is found in whole grain breads and cereals, fruits and vegetables, legumes, nuts, and seeds. Fiber comes in two forms: soluble and insoluble. For maximum health benefits from fiber, it is important to eat both forms of fiber on a regular basis.

Soluble fiber is found in oat bran and in dried beans and peas—including kidney beans, lentils and chick peas—as well as in many fruits and vegetables. Soluble fiber is helpful as a natural cholesterol-lowering agent, as an aid to slowing the absorption of sugar and thus helping in the fight against diabetes, and in reducing the risk of developing gallstones.

Insoluble fiber, the type of fiber found in whole grains, nuts, seeds, and a whole slew of fruits and vegetables, is nature's perfect defense mechanism against colon cancer. As a natural sponge, insoluble fiber soaks up water from the large intestine and gains bulk. The bulkiness of this fiber combines with other waste products and rapidly carries them through your intestines. In this way, toxins and other potential cancer-causing chemicals are flushed out of your body before they begin causing health problems.

Insoluble fiber also helps in the prevention of constipation. You may never suffer from hemorrhoids again if you get your fair share of this fiber—and drink lots of water. Without adequate water in your system, that spongy fiber can get bound up in your bowels and result in tough stools that may be difficult to pass.

Both types of fiber share a natural ability to cause a pleasant sensation of satiety. As fiber moves through our gut and swells, it produces a sensation of fullness in our belly. The full feeling we experience after eating foods rich in fiber can be a godsend to those who are trying to lose weight.

So let's eat fiber, nature's multipurpose bowel cleanser, cholesterol-lowering agent, cancer-fighter, and natural satiety-inducer. One of the tastiest ways we know to increase your fiber intake is by eating fruits and vegetables.

It is easy for us to relish the taste of a juicy red apple or the sweet and refreshing sensation of biting into a ripe watermelon. Still, as a society we consume far less fruit on a daily basis than we should. Surveys show that the average American eats less than two fruit servings per day.

A fruit serving can be as simple as a six-ounce glass of orange juice, a medium-sized fruit such as an apple or pear, a quarter of a small cantaloupe, half a cup of canned fruit, or half a grapefruit. An easy way to meet your recommended servings of up to four fruits per day is to eat fruit as snacks or desserts. Try it!

These days people in general look upon fruits as boring. What is exciting about eating an apple or peeling and biting off a piece of a banana? What would your fellow workers think if you brought a plain old plum or peach to work for your snack? Who would be impressed if you brought a large bowl of fruit cocktail to your next work party?

Were fruits always this boring? No! Did you ever stop to think how much fruits were revered by our ancestors a little over one hundred years ago? In 1894, the master impressionist painter Paul Cezanne completed his now famous painting "La Corbeille De Pommes" (Basket of Apples). Painting fruit as still life became an obsession for many artists.

Today our society has apparently lost its awe of fruits. Fruit is used mostly for fancy displays at buffets and parties, or as a garnish to a carefully prepared meal. Instead of admiring the fantastic array of fruit on the table or on our plates, we should be eating them!

One fruit that has come to symbolize the epitome of good health is the apple. Made popular by the legendary "Johnny Appleseed" in the early nineteenth century, the apple has come a long way from its reputation in earlier life as the forbidden fruit in the Garden of Eden.

With many varieties and different shades of red, yellow, green, and combinations of these colors, the apple is visually appealing to all who enjoy it. The soft, shiny, and polishable skin of the apple belies its head-turning unique crunchiness on the inside.

Taking a bite out of a juicy and delectable apple represents an ability to savor life to its fullest. The experience is life-affirming and refreshing. So, go ahead and sink your teeth into a golden green or bright red apple. It might be the best prescription for good health your doctor will never write!

Sophie and I have included below brief descriptions of many fruits and vegetables. Accompanying the descriptions are some interesting facts about each item. Enjoy!

Fruits and vegetables: a sampling

Apple: The best-known and most popular grown fruit. Even though the apple came to North America as an immigrant, it has become a typical American product, lending itself to the popular phrase, "as American as apple pie." There are over 7,000 varieties of apples grown in the world. More than 2,500 of these varieties are grown in the United States. Some of the most highly regarded kinds include Cortland, Golden Delicious, Granny Smith, and McIntosh.

Asparagus: Comes in two forms: 1) a tasty green vegetable and 2) an ornamental plant. A delicate but savory vegetable, asparagus was first grown on land bordering the Mediterranean Sea. The ancient Greeks and Romans used asparagus for food and medicine. It is a good source of folic acid.

Banana: Originally found in Asian countries, the banana now grows in tropical countries throughout the world. Brazil is the leading banana producer. Rich in potassium, it is one of nature's healthiest snacks.

Brussels Sprouts: Each sprout looks like a tiny head of cabbage. Brussels sprouts undoubtedly are of Belgian origin. They are a good source of vitamins A and C.

Cantaloupe: Member of the muskmelon family and cousin to the honeydew melon. Its name is derived from the town of Cantaloupo, Italy. Rich in vitamins A and C, it is a good source of potassium, too.

Carrot: Made famous by Mel Blanc's cartoon character Bugs Bunny, a carrot is easy to eat in salads, steamed as part of a cooked meal, or enjoyed all on its own. The versatile carrot is extremely rich in a group of substances called carotenes. Beta carotenes, the best known carotenes, are the precursors to vitamin A. The carrot has been a staple of the North American diet for generations and will surely always have a place on our dinner tables.

Cauliflower: Well-known for its head of tightly clustered flowers. Cauliflower resembles broccoli in that they both offer a selection of crunchy vegetable pieces that remind you of a floral bouquet while at the same time providing you with a good source of vitamin C.

Kale: A relatively obscure vegetable, kale is a well-rounded vegetable in that it supplies a strong amount of vitamins A, C, K, as well as calcium, and good amounts of many other vitamins and minerals. Like brussels sprouts, kale is a member of the cabbage family.

Kiwi: Named after the shaggy, flightless bird that is a native of New Zealand, the kiwi is a soft, edible fruit that has grown in popularity over the last two decades. Kiwis ripen slowly but are well worth the wait. Furry on the outside, the kiwi boasts a green and sparkling inside that is a pleasure to look at and a delight to eat.

Leek: Familiar to you if you have ever enjoyed leek soup, this vegetable bares a mild resemblance to the green onion. Popular in Wales, United Kingdom, leeks can be boiled and served alone, or included in soups and stews.

Mango: About the size of a large apple, but weighing considerably more. The mango consists of a soft, juicy, yellow or orange pulp covered by skin that may be either yellow, red, or green. Mangoes are usually shaped like a kidney, but may be round or egg-shaped. This dense tropical fruit is the best fruit source of vitamin A.

Mushroom: Of the roughly 38,000 known species of mushrooms, only about 1,000 of them are safe to eat. Edible mushrooms can be eaten creamed, baked, fried, broiled, stewed, or served in salads. Mushrooms are eaten throughout the world and are considered a delicacy in a few countries. One piece of advice: do not pick your own mushrooms—some are deadly!

Peach: Second only to the apple in distribution throughout the world. More peaches are grown in the United States than in all other countries combined. The peach is similar in every way to the nectarine except in the texture of its skin. If you are ever in Georgia, do not forget to have a bowl of peaches and cream (less cream, more peaches!) on one of the dozens of Peachtree streets in that state.

Pear: Its shape is unmistakable: large and round at the bottom and tapering inward toward its stem. The pear's juicy flesh is sweet and mellow. The pear is a close cousin to the apple: 1) the pear tree resembles the apple tree; 2) pears are nutritionally similar to apples; and 3) a pear's seedy core is much like the core of an apple. However, the one intangible difference between them is that the pear has never been as popular as the apple!

Peppers: You have two choices of peppers: mild and sweet *bell peppers,* named for their bell-like shape, and hot *chili peppers,* naturally spicy due to their fiery ingredient capsaicin. Green peppers are great snacks all by themselves or eaten with your favorite dip. Stuffing green peppers can be a fun family activity when preparing a meal and may inject some enthusiasm into your child's appetite for this healthy vegetable. One pepper contains an entire day's worth of vitamin C!

Plum: Easy to eat, the plum may be as small as a cherry or as large as a small peach. Its shape may be round or oval. The thin skin may be green, yellow, red, blue, or purple. Some plums can be enjoyed on their own; others are used to make jelly, preserves, plum butter, and jam.

Potato: Best grown and harvested in cooler climates, the potato is a popular and versatile vegetable. Adopted by the Irish as their main food in the eighteenth and nineteenth centuries, the potato is now a worldly vegetable. All fifty states grow the potato commercially as do many countries throughout the world. Sophie and I haven't found a potato yet that we did not like!

Pumpkin: A super source of vitamin A, the pumpkin has become a symbol of autumn. At Halloween, pumpkins are carved into jack-o'-lanterns. Pumpkin pie is a family tradition for Thanksgiving Dinner.

Spinach: Spinach is a great vegetable to eat. Its sweet leaves go well in salads or cooked as a side dish. The comic strip character Popeye knew the value of spinach. It is loaded with many vitamins and minerals, especially iron.

Tomato: The tomato is probably the most useful garden product for our eating pleasure. Juicy when ripe, the tomato is a fixture in our North American diet. Also referred to as the "love apple," the tomato's aphrodisiac superstitions are widely known. Lycopene, a phytochemical recently shown to play a role in reducing the risk of developing certain cancers, is found in abundance in tomatoes.

Watermelon: A classic hot summer's day fruit, a succulent and refreshing watermelon brings us a cool taste that can perk up even the laziest summer day. One question about a watermelon that is still up for debate: Should you swallow its seeds? Whatever your preference, happiness is enjoying the fruity feeling of a watermelon in season!

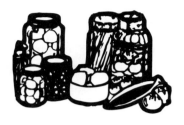

The Miracle Foods, Part 3

Chapter 8

Vitamins and Minerals

"Good things come in small packages."
Anonymous

THE HUMAN BODY IS A COLLECTION of many different systems, each with its unique function, purpose, and needs. Our bodies could not survive without the presence of the following systems: circulatory, respiratory, gastrointestinal, genito-urinary, musculoskeletal, neurological, and others. In plain English, we could not live if we did not have a heart, lungs, stomach and intestines, kidneys and sex organs, bones, and all the rest.

Given the complexity of the human body and the constant maintenance and repairs going on inside our bodies throughout every day of our lives, I find it amazing that we depend on microscopic amounts of substances like vitamins and minerals for our well-being. Even more fascinating is that without these trace amounts of "vital amines" and minerals on a daily basis, our bodies begin to run less efficiently, and eventually display signs of disease. We need vitamins and minerals for our very survival!

Oh, yes, let's not forget. There is something else we need every day in order to function: water, water, and more water!

Most of us are guilty of not drinking an adequate supply of water. Our bodies are 90 percent water by volume. All of our tissues are bathed every second in fluid, of which water is the major component. Without water it takes only three days for our bodies to literally "dry up" from within and then we die! Think of it. Only three days! Water is the ultimate prerequisite for good health.

Vitamins and minerals work in our bodies at the cellular level, the smallest level within the marvelously sophisticated machine we call the human body. As you are reading these words, chemical and biological reactions of vital importance are going on inside every living cell of your body.

These complex biochemical reactions help run your body's internal engine. Thousands of these reactions take place every minute of your life. And guess what? All of these intricate reactions are interlinked with one another. You need to have one reaction occur for the next one to happen, and so forth. Take away even one of these precious reactions and a link has been lost in the chain of your body's mystifying order of things. Theoretically, it is possible to bypass or circumvent a missing reaction, but practically speaking, this does not happen.

As we approach the beginning of the twenty-first century, vitamins and minerals are rapidly becoming the focus of our attention in our human quest to live healthier and longer. Can vitamins and minerals help us achieve these goals?

This book is not meant to answer the above question. There are plenty of good resource books and publications which try to answer, both directly and indirectly, the all-important question of whether or not vitamins and minerals can improve and prolong our lives. This

VITAMINS AND MINERALS

particular chapter is presented to help increase your awareness of food sources rich in vitamins and minerals.

Our modern way of life brings us pleasures far beyond what most humans dreamed of in the past. Our way of life is too comfortable for our own good! We don't exercise or do physical labor nearly as much as we useed to only a few decades ago.

Our luxuries have given us more time for leisure and have freed up our time for interesting pursuits. Our eating habits, however, have suffered as a result of all this modernization. We no longer need to go out and plant, hunt and harvest our own food with our bare hands. With modern technology, food is grown, picked, processed, packaged, and transported to our local supermarkets and grocery stores without inconveniencing us. All it takes is a short ride to the store to get almost anything we desire. Restaurants also cater to our every culinary whim, freeing us from the chores of preparing foods in our kitchens.

There is one thing, however, you cannot order by telephone or get at your local store or restaurant. It is the most elusive and earnestly sought after commodity in the entire world. This ideal: **good health**.

How do you go about getting good health? You can't buy it. Or can you?

Millions of Americans are taking nutritional or dietary supplements every day in their search for better health. Are you one of them? Who doesn't want to have good health? If you believed there was a sure way to obtain good health, you would try it, wouldn't you? Well, hundreds of edible products (foods!) are available that have been tried and tested over and over. Their ability to improve your overall well-being and help your body to perform at its best has been proven beyond reasonable doubt.

Among the hundreds of healthful foods, we have focused our attention in the preceding chapters (see chapters 6 and 7) on nature's most colorful and valuable foods: fruits and vegetables.

No other foods do a better job of providing the recommended and required daily doses of the microscopic amounts of vitamins and minerals your body needs for better health than do fruits and vegetables.

Yes, you may think you need to take a daily vitamin and mineral supplement if you are not certain about your food choices for the day. Some may argue that it would be wise to take a vitamin and mineral supplement on a daily basis. So, why don't all of us take supplements?

Here's a simple answer. Vitamins are like drugs. In appropriate amounts they can work wonders for our health. However, too much of a good thing is no good. Vitamins and minerals taken in excessive amounts are eliminated by our bodies in the urine and feces. When we take in more vitamins or minerals than we need, it is wasted—literally. All the water-soluble vitamins and minerals are flushed out of our bodies by the kidneys and down the toilet. Americans probably have the world's most expensive urine!

Not all vitamins and minerals are discarded on a daily basis. Some are stored in our fat stores for safe keeping. Others are hidden away in our bones, hair, and any other storage place our body deems necessary. Toxic levels can build up quickly if mega doses of our tiny vitamin and mineral friends are ingested too frequently.

Of course, people with certain medical conditions may need to take vitamin or mineral supplements in order to maintain normal function. Cystic fibrosis, osteoporosis, iron deficiency, and anemia are examples of such health problems. Other conditions require an extra dose of a particular vitamin or mineral for scientifically proven reasons. For example, folic acid supplementation before and during pregnancy can help prevent brain and spinal cord problems in a newborn.

In this part of the chapter, we will give you a brief description of the roles of key vitamins and minerals as well as hints about where you can find each of these biochemical players in the foods you choose to eat. Not all of the vitamins and minerals are mentioned here, just a sampling.

By enticing you with a handful of facts on selected vitamins and minerals, we hope to encourage further discussion and exploration on your part to better understand the value of these wonderful micronutrients. And remember, the best source of these miniature biochemical actors is found in the foods you eat. Enjoy!

Below are some of the most commonly mentioned vitamins and minerals in today's health circles. We list them in random order, not by their importance. We allude only to the best-known functions and food sources. We have omitted references to RDA (Recommended Dietary Allowance) as well as toxic doses. Occasional mention of deficiency states of a particular vitamin or mineral has been included. Additional resources for information about vitamins and minerals are included in the recommended reading list at the end of this book.

Vitamins

Vitamin A

The first vitamin discovered, vitamin A plays many roles in maintaining our body, the most notable one that of preserving night vision. Vitamin A is needed to make "visual purple," the eye pigment responsible for proper vision when light is limited. Without sufficient amounts of vitamin A in the body, night blindness may result. Other roles of vitamin A include assuring the integrity of the skin and keeping the lining of the gastrointestinal and respiratory tracts smooth and trouble free. Normal growth and reproduction also depend upon adequate amount of vitamin A.

Vitamin A is fat soluble and comes in two forms: preformed vitamin A, or retinol, and provitamin A, known as carotene. Beta carotene, the best-known precursor of vitamin A, is one of the best antioxidants available to the body. Vitamin A comes from both animal and plant sources. Major animal-derived food sources of Vitamin A include liver, egg yolk, cheese, milk, and butter. Major plant sources include dark orange and yellow fruits and vegetables such as apricots, cantaloupe, carrots, mangoes, pumpkins, and sweet potatoes; and dark green and leafy vegetables such as asparagus, spinach, or broccoli.

Vitamin B1 (Thiamine)

Vitamin B1, or thiamine, was discovered in 1934 by chemist Robert Williams. A thiamine deficiency can be deadly. Also known as beriberi, thiamine deficiency was first attributed to eating a diet consisting chiefly of polished rice or refined wheat. Beriberi is now rare in the Western world, except among alcoholics and people who make poor food choices through ignorance, poverty, or neglect. Beriberi may lead to neurological damage and heart failure.

Thiamine is water soluble and needs to be replenished daily. This vitamin plays a key role in nerve function and is an important biological catalyst for many biochemical reactions in the body.

Best sources of thiamine include pork, organ meats, whole grains, wheat germ, and enriched breads and cereals.

Vitamin B2 (Riboflavin)

Named for its rich yellow color (from the Latin word flavius, meaning "yellow"), riboflavin plays an active role in energy metabolism. Like other B vitamins, it is not stored in the body and must be replaced daily through consumption of nutritious foods.

Riboflavin is found in animal protein sources such as eggs, meat, fish, poultry, liver, and milk and dairy products such as yogurt and cheese. Milk is the best source of riboflavin in the American diet. Other sources include dark green and leafy vegetables, and enriched breads and cereals.

Pantothenic Acid (formerly Vitamin B3)

Named for its ubiquitous nature, (from the Greek word *pantos*, meaning "everywhere") pantothenic acid is found in all foods. This vitamin plays a role in the release of energy from carbohydrates, fats, and proteins.

The best sources of pantothenic acid are eggs, salmon, organ meats, peanuts, wheat bran, brewer's yeast, and almost every vegetable.

Vitamin B6 (Pyridoxine)

Vitamin B6 is present in all foods in one of three forms: pyridoxine, pyridoxamine, or pyridoxal (not to be confused with "paradoxical"!) This vitamin is essential for the conversion of tryptophan (an important amino acid) into niacin (see below). Vitamin B6 also helps with protein metabolism.

Pyridoxine is found in all foods in varying degrees. The best food sources include liver, pork, legumes (dried beans and peas), wheat germ, whole grains, brewer's yeast, bananas, and potatoes.

Niacin

Niacin is best known as the nutrient responsible for preventing pellagra. Pellagra is a disease in which a person suffers from four Ds: Dermatitis, a scaling and dry skin; Diarrhea; Disorientation; and Death. Niacin is like the other B vitamins in that it plays an active role in the metabolism of proteins, carbohydrates, and fats. When niacin is prescribed in the form of nicotinic acid in high doses, it can lower your cholesterol. However, severe facial flushing, a temporary yet possibly uncomfortable sensation, often results following ingestion of this form of niacin.

Major sources of niacin include meat, fish, poultry, organ meats, eggs, peanuts, legumes, and brewer's yeast.

Folate

Also known as folacin and folic acid, folate provides a vital function in the making of the blueprint of life: DNA (DeoxyriboNucleicAcid). Therefore, folate helps in the production of new cells throughout the entire body. An inadequate intake of folate within the first few weeks of pregnancy has been linked to brain and spinal cord problems in the unborn child.

Folate derives its name from the word foliage, implying plant life. Not surprisingly, the best sources of folate include green and leafy vegetables like asparagus, broccoli, spinach, and romaine lettuce, as well as oranges, whole grain breads and cereals, liver, nuts, and legumes.

Vitamin B12 (Cobalamin)

Available commercially as cyanocobalamin, vitamin B12 is supplied exclusively in our diet from animal sources. Strict vegetarians may need to take vitamin B12 supplements to reduce the risk of pernicious anemia (anemia in which the body experiences widespread nerve damage). Among other functions, vitamin B12—

a) helps to form and regenerate red blood cells,

b) maintains the health of our nervous system,

c) aids in the absorption of folate.

Meat, poultry, fish, organ meats, eggs, cheese, and milk are all good sources of vitamin B12.

Vitamin C (Ascorbic Acid)

An antioxidant protects other substances from being damaged by oxygen. Vitamin C, one of the best antioxidant vitamins, has become famous due to the efforts of the scientist Dr. Linus Pauling. Pauling, who lived into his 90s, espoused doses of vitamin C far in excess of what a normal human can acquire naturally from foods. Pauling did not definitively prove that supplemental mega doses of vitamin C cured or prevented any disease. However, his good health and long life helped link his name forever with vitamin C.

You have probably heard that sailors during the sixteenth and seventeenth centuries suffered from scurvy, the scourge of seamen. When limes were distributed to sailors on the open sea scurvy was all but eliminated. Vitamin C, also known as ascorbic acid (meaning "without scurvy") was officially discovered in the 1930s.

Citrus fruits and their juices such as oranges, grapefruits, lemons, and limes are excellent sources of vitamin C. Many other fresh fruits and vegetables supply vitamin C, including bell peppers, broccoli, brussels sprouts, cabbage, cantaloupe, mangoes, spinach, strawberries, tangerines, tomatoes, papayas, potatoes, and more. Rosehips from rose bushes are also rich in "the sunshine vitamin," lending credence to rose-hip tea as a nutritious beverage.

Minerals

Calcium

The most abundant mineral in the human body, calcium is needed regularly in adequate amounts to develop and maintain strong bones. Since our bones are constantly being molded and remolded (not that we can feel it!), we need a daily supply of calcium to maintain our skeleton. Consuming food sources rich in calcium can help us to stave off bone diseases such as osteoporosis, osteomalacia, and rickets. These three diseases are directly related to either improper usage or lack of calcium in the body. Calcium is second only to iron as the most common mineral deficiency in the diet of American women.

The best source of calcium is a big glass of milk, preferably skim milk if you are watching your waistline. Vitamin D added to milk during pasteurization and homogenization increases the body's absorption of calcium. Skim milk also contains slightly more calcium than the higher fat milks on the market. Drinking just two 8-ounce glasses of milk a day will supply half the calcium most people need for a lifetime of healthy bones.

If you suffer from lactose intolerance and cannot drink lactose-free milk, you will need to seek out other sources of dietary calcium to avoid developing brittle bones. Other calcium sources include yogurt, cheese, dark green and leafy vegetables, nuts, seeds, fish bones found in sardines and salmon, tofu (with calcium added in processing), and more recently, calcium-fortified juices.

Phosphorus

Along with calcium, phosphorus is essential for healthy bones and teeth. You need as much phosphorus as you do calcium in your diet. Luckily, phosphorus is found in most foods.

The best sources are milk, meat, poultry, fish, eggs, whole grains, nuts, and legumes.

Potassium

A major role for potassium is modulating nerve impulse transmission so that our muscles receive the messages from our brain in a coordinated fashion. Other important functions include regulating the heart rhythm and helping to maintain proper fluid balance throughout the body.

Potassium's best sources are a variety of fruits and vegetables such as bananas, cantaloupe, honeydew melon, oranges, dried fruits, tomatoes, potatoes, as well as milk, and meat.

Magnesium

Magnesium is required in over 300 known biochemical reactions in the body. Available in hard water, magnesium is also found in most foods.

The best food sources of magnesium are nuts, whole grains, green vegetables, and legumes.

Sodium

Sodium is necessary for life. Part of the common and naturally occurring compound we know as salt (sodium chloride), sodium is easily consumed in excess of our bodily needs. The average American eats almost ten times the daily requirement of sodium every day. This is because salt is used extensively in processing foods to permit longer shelf-life and storage of our foods. Avoiding the salt shaker has become a common custom among people afflicted with high blood pressure (hypertension). Millions of Americans suffer from hypertension, with many people going on to develop strokes, heart attacks, and kidney failure as a result. Sodium should not be shrugged off as just another mineral.

Sodium is found in many foods. Canned foods and frozen dinners contain significantly more sodium than fresh foods. Other notable contributors of sodium to our diet include salt, processed foods, deli foods, snack foods such as potato chips, and condiments such as soy sauce, mustard, relish, and ketchup.

Zinc

Zinc is a metallic mineral that our bodies need for a variety of functions, including 1) proper growth of skin, hair, and nails; 2) normal operation of a man's prostate gland; and 3) efficient use of the body's insulin, the hormone chiefly responsible for regulating and controlling the level of blood sugar.

More recently, zinc lozenges have been promoted as an aid to fighting off the common cold. Whether or not zinc lozenges help you recover faster from a cold, they are not recommended as a dietary source of zinc.

Oysters contain the most concentrated source of zinc. Zinc is also found in meat, poultry, liver, and eggs. Whole grain products, too, contain fair amounts of this alphabetically challenged mineral.

Iron

The most common vitamin/mineral deficiency worldwide is iron deficiency. Approximately 8 percent of women in the United States have symptoms of iron deficiency. Because so much of the body's iron is found in the blood, women are more likely to suffer from lower iron levels than men due to women's regular monthly loss of blood through menstruation.

Without adequate iron, we cannot perform at peak efficiency. Many people, especially women, feel they should take iron supplements to make up for their low iron levels. This may lead to an iron overload.

There are two kinds of iron overload. One is inherited and the other is caused by ingesting too much iron in supplements. The hereditary condition, hemochromatosis, causes the body's level of iron to rise to dangerous levels that can lead to multi-organ disease and possible death. Whether caused by diet or heredity, iron toxicity in the body is noted by symptoms such as severe nausea, vomiting, abdominal pain, diarrhea, and feelings of weakness. Extreme toxicity can be fatal. Be careful not to overuse iron supplements.

Iron in food is available in two forms: heme and non-heme. Of the two, heme iron is more easily absorbed by the body and is found principally in meat, liver, poultry, and fish. Non-heme iron is found in vegetable and plant sources such as legumes, dark green and leafy vegetables, dark molasses, dried fruits, and whole grains.

Iron absorption is enhanced by combining a food source rich in vitamin C (such as orange juice or a citrus fruit) with or after your meal. Certain substances may decrease iron absorption. Tannins, which are found naturally in teas, combine with the iron and prevent it from being absorbed. To maximize iron absorption, it is wise to wait at least an hour following your meal before enjoying your favorite tea. Antacids and calcium supplements with a calcium carbonate base, when taken at meal time, may also inhibit iron absorption. The best time to take these supplements is between meals or at bedtime.

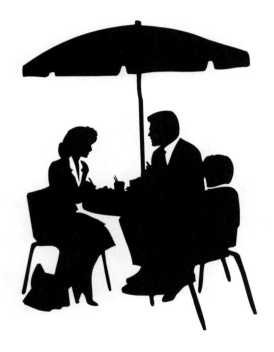

Chapter 9

Mood for Food

"Since childhood, I've dealt with stress by keeping to myself, reading books, and eating anything and everything I could find!"
Anonymous

ARE YOU ALWAYS IN THE MOOD for food? Do you ever consider the reasons why you are in the mood for food? Do you eat in response to your emotional state, to stress, to environmental or social situations? What triggers you to eat?

The answers to these questions can help you become more aware of how you relate to food. Each of us has a very personal relationship with food. We share intimate moments with food. Food is with us through good times and bad times, from birth to old age, in our greatest and saddest moments in life. Birthdays, weddings, births, funerals, parties and celebrations of all kinds center around food. We attach our emotions and our memories to food.

Food is much more than its caloric and nutritional value; it is rich with life. As we learn to deal with life, we must also learn to deal with food. Just like it is important to understand a friend or family member, it is also important to understand food. Food should become our friend. Instead of viewing food as a weight-gaining product and our enemy, we should embrace food and learn the ways it affects us, as well as how our own behaviors, emotions, and thoughts all affect our interaction with food.

To help you better understand your eating style, take a few moments to check off which of these statements, listed below, applies to you. (Table 1)

Table 1

Eating Style: Conditioned Eating vs Emotional Eating

Section A: Conditioned Eating

☐ I eat fast

☐ I eat the leftovers

☐ I often take second helpings

☐ I end my meal with a dessert

☐ I eat while I am cooking

☐ I hide to eat

☐ I eat until I get sick

☐ I wake up at night to eat

☐ I eat when I see others eat

☐ I eat too much on special occasions

☐ I am always or often thinking of food

MOOD FOR FOOD

☐ I eat because it is time to eat

☐ I use food as a reward

☐ I snack on foods while watching TV

☐ I eat so as not to disappoint the hostess

☐ _____

☐ _____

Section B: Emotional Eating

☐ I eat for fear of being hungry later

☐ I eat when I am bored

☐ I eat when I am anxious

☐ I eat when I am nervous

☐ I eat when I am happy

☐ I eat when I am sad

☐ I eat when I am frustrated

☐ I eat when I am lonely

☐ I eat when I am stressed

☐ I eat when I cry

☐ _____

☐ _____

Can you think of any other emotions, behaviors, thoughts, or situations that may provoke you to eat? If so, add them to the list.

Statements found in both Section A and Section B are a result of what is referred to as false hunger. False hunger encompasses both emotional and conditioned eating. Statements in Section A of Table 1 are a result of what is referred to as **conditioned eating**. Those who exhibit this type of eating are called "conditioned" eaters.

Conditioned eaters do not listen to their bodies. Instead, they eat in response to certain experiences, events, or situations—for example, eating because it is time to eat or eating as a reward. Conditioned eating occurs in response to external cues such as watching a mouth-watering television food commercial, noting a particular time on the clock, seeing others eat, or the sight of food itself. An external cue can trigger the desire to eat in someone who is experiencing a false hunger.

False hunger also involves what is referred to as **emotional eating** as illustrated by examples in Section B of Table 1. People who exhibit this type of eating are referred to as "emotional" eaters. Emotional eaters "eat their emotions." Any emotion may dictate what these individuals eat, regardless of whether or not they are physiologically hungry. Emotional eaters use the act of eating to distract themselves from their emotional state. For example, they will eat during or following a stressful event instead of dealing with the stressful event itself.

The major difference between emotional and conditioned eating is that emotional eating deals strictly with emotions that lead to food intake, while conditioned eating is associated with eating in response to external cues, events, experiences, and situations.

To classify yourself accurately as an emotional and/or conditioned eater, you must first be experiencing an impairment in your normal functioning—regardless of how many statements you have checked in Table 1. If you are unable to attend to your daily activities because of distracting thoughts of food or preoccupation concerning food intake, this would classify you as an emotional and/or conditioned eater.

Conditioned eaters and emotional eaters have lost their innate ability to listen to and decipher their internal physiological body cues.

What leads these people to neglect their body signals or internal cues? Among the many reasons, a common thread that links people with the above eating habits is our society's fast-paced lifestyle. These individuals do not have nor make the time to focus on their bodies. Society has adopted a "fix-it-quick" mentality. Eating a food item in response to stress, for example, may be more gratifying in the very-short term compared to dealing with the stress itself and the issues surrounding the stressful situation.

These eating behaviors may become a habit. As you know, it takes effort, motivation, and willingness to modify a habit. Individuals who experience false hunger have become stuck in the way they deal with their hunger. I will share some effective ways to deal with false hunger a little later in the chapter.

As stated above, both emotional and conditioned eaters have a difficult time sensing true physiological hunger symptoms related to a drop in blood sugar, such as light-headedness, difficulty concentrating, queasiness, restlessness, and don't forget the rumbling stomach! These symptoms may vary from person to person. The only way to start "re-listening" to your internal body cues is to be able to distinguish between false hunger and true hunger. First, you need to understand what true hunger is all about.

True hunger occurs when your body is *physiologically* (not psychologically) in need of food energy in the form of calories. One way to determine if you are experiencing a true hunger is to "listen" to your body and take note of your body's physical responses as listed above in order to realize their significance.

Another way to identify true hunger is to recall the time of your last meal or snack. Suppose you've just enjoyed a 100-200 calorie snack. In theory, it will take about an hour for your body to burn off all the calories derived from that snack. Only then will you start to experience true hunger.

Using the same concept, the energy derived from a meal would require more time to be burned off by your body. So, allow your body about three hours to burn off the calories derived from a 400-600 calorie meal. A rule of thumb is to allow about one hour to elapse for every 100 to 200 calories of energy consumed.

It is important to "listen" to your body and feel the hunger before enjoying your next meal or snack. This true physiological hunger is a sign that your body has indeed finished burning off the calories from your last meal or snack and is ready for more. Careful attention to your body's internal cues will help you recognize true hunger and can help keep you from eating too much and too often.

The quality of the food is as important as the timing of the food intake. Choosing the right foods to eat at meals and snacks is key. To learn the principles of sound nutrition, go back to basics. To refresh your memory of the United States Department of Agriculture (USDA) Food Guide Pyramid, see Chapter 4, Figure 1.

True hunger is easier to deal with than false hunger because true hunger requires responding to a physiological symptom in the form of food. False hunger, on the other hand, involves multiple variables including emotions, experiences, thoughts, events, or situations which can all trigger a desire to eat.

How does one differentiate a true hunger from a false hunger? One way to distinguish between these two types of hunger is to verbally ask yourself out loud whether you are experiencing a true hunger or a false hunger. I recommend **out loud**, as the sound of your own voice can be a powerful tool for increasing your awareness.

The next time you feel hungry, ask yourself out loud, "Is this a false hunger or a true hunger?" Once you know you are experiencing true hunger, go ahead and eat, confident in the knowledge that your body is truly in need of food.

On the other hand, to verify that you are experiencing a false hunger, you need to identify and determine the emotion that is tempting you to eat. To do this, it is essential to become comfortable with the entire gamut of emotions ranging from happiness to sadness, excitement to boredom, etc. The ability to pinpoint an emotion that may lead you to eat is key in dealing with false hunger. Table 2 (following page) is included to help you become more aware of your emotions. Ask yourself how you would react to each of the following emotions and note which ones stimulate your desire to eat:

Table 2: Identification of Emotions

HOW DO YOU REACT TO—	
anger	
boredom	
discouragement	
excitement	
frustration	
guilt	
happiness	
helplessness	
indecisiveness	
irritability	
loneliness	
panic	
rejection	
remorse	
sadness	
stress	

Just as it is important to identify emotions that can influence you to eat, it is also important to identify external cues. Included below in Table 3 is a list of common external cues that may provoke eating. Can you think of other situations, events, objects, thoughts, or places which may tempt you to eat? If so write them down. Indicate how you would react to each of the following and note which ones stimulate your desire to eat.

Table 3: Identification of External Cues

HOW DO YOU REACT TO—	
a certain room in your home	
a certain memory	
a smell/odor/fragrance	
a song heard on the radio	
half-full refrigerator	
half-empty refrigerator	
a certain beverage	
a school lunch bell	
television commercials	
sight of food	
a particular time on the clock	

External cues gathered by our five external senses—seeing, hearing, smelling, touching, and tasting—help us interact with the world around us. For many of us, our sensory input directs us to eat even though our internal alarm clock has not signaled us to do so. Who can resist the sights, smells, or sounds of a favorite food being prepared for our eating pleasure even though we may not truly need to eat? Seeing food ads in magazines or on television, smelling the aroma of freshly baked bread or mom's hot apple pie, or hearing a conversation about your favorite food are examples of familiar external eating cues.

The above sensations can result in irresistible urges to eat no matter what our internal hunger level may be. External cues start the flow of saliva and stomach acids, simulating the sensation of hunger. Internal cues are more subtle, but truer in the sense that your body is letting you know it is time to eat: feeling less energetic or more sluggish, a hunger pang in your belly, perhaps even a mild headache. You may experience slight variations in how your body's internal cues tell you it is time to eat.

Your job is to know your body so that you can feel the messages your body is sending and know how to respond. Only then will you learn to feed your body at the appropriate times.

Once you have identified the emotions and external cues that tempt you to eat, ask yourself why you turn to certain foods in response to your external cues or emotions.

Try to understand exactly what triggered a given emotion or cue. Was it an event, a situation, an experience, or a place that led you to experience false hunger? To help increase your awareness of your relationship with food, take a moment to jot down some of your emotions or other common external cues that lead you to eat. (See Table 4.) Note what triggered that particular emotion or external cue. Leave blank the "alternate action" column for now. Consider the following examples:

Table 4: Identifying Your Hunger Triggers

EMOTION or EXTERNAL CUE	TRIGGER (event, person, situation, place)	ALTERNATE ACTION (in place of eating)
boredom (emotion)	finished my work day	opening mail
walking by the ice-cream stand (external cue)	at the mall	walk into magazine shop

Eating is an activity like walking, studying, reading, and house cleaning. If you experience false hunger, it is crucial for you to think of alternate activities you can do rather than the activity of eating. Coming up with a plan of action that is realistic for you is imperative. Your plan of action can include not only sporting or exercise activities, but also work-related activities, house-related activities, or pleasurable activities.

The following Activity Table (Table 5) is divided into "necessary activities" and "leisurely activities."

Add activities of your own that apply to your specific needs and are compatible with your lifestyle.

Table 5: Identification of Activities

Necessary Activities
Vacuuming
Washing dishes
Walking the dog
Cleaning the bird cage
Doing a load of laundry
Leisurely Activities
Listening to music
Reading a book
Taking a walk
Taking a bath
Going to the mall
Riding a bike
Writing in a journal
Telephoning a friend or family member
Meditating

Now go back to Table 4 and complete the "alternate action" column. For each emotion or external cue, think of an activity you can do other than eating during those times in which you are experiencing false hunger. Don't despair! False hunger will eventually subside, but it will subside even quicker if you are distracted or involved in an activity.

Sometimes it will feel as if it is next to impossible to fight off your false hunger. You will feel compelled to submit to your craving for the food item. If you must, *give yourself permission* to do so. This is an important concept—allowing yourself to eat. If you sincerely give yourself permission to eat, you will see your desire for that food dwindle over time, and you will be less inclined to overindulge in the particular food item you've had your heart set on.

If you question the above, ask yourself: have you ever craved oranges, celery, or bell peppers? Probably not! This is because we give ourselves permission to eat as many fruits and vegetables as we can. You want to approach the foods you crave (when experiencing a false hunger) in the same way you relate to fruits and vegetables.

Giving yourself permission to eat means there will be no guilt associated with that "forbidden" food item. However, it should not lead to eating whatever you want, whenever you want, in whatever quantity. You still want to be sensitive to your sense of hunger and take appropriate actions to deal with the type of hunger you are experiencing.

In addition to giving yourself permission to eating a particular food, it is important to know how to enjoy that food item to the absolute fullest. If done correctly, you will not eat as much.

Here is what I mean. First, look at the food. Notice the color, texture and any other features about that food item which strikes you. Then, take a big deep breath in through your nose, all the while appreciating the food's aromatic presence. Following your first bite, be sure to chew well so that all of your taste buds can appreciate and savor all the different flavors. The last step is to swallow your food.

This sequence of events can be done with every bite and may take up to five minutes. As the food is swallowed, note that the chewed food is no longer tasted nor appreciated. That is why we're always impatient for the next bite!

Just as it is important to become familiar with all of your emotions and external cues which may provoke a sense of false hunger, it is also worthwhile to become fully aware of "problem" foods that may lead to overeating. Consider the list of foods below in Table 6, checking off all foods that pose a problem for you.

Table 6: Possible Problem Foods

Grain group
- ❑ Bread
- ❑ Cereal
- ❑ Rice
- ❑ Pasta
- ❑ Crackers
- ❑ _____

Dairy group
- ❑ Milk
- ❑ Chocolate milk
- ❑ Yogurt
- ❑ Cheese
- ❑ _____

Bakery group
- ❑ Muffins
- ❑ Donuts
- ❑ Cakes
- ❑ Pies
- ❑ Cookies
- ❑ Croissants
- ❑ _____

Beverage group
- ❑ Water
- ❑ Juice
- ❑ Sodas
- ❑ Tea
- ❑ Coffee
- ❑ Alcohol
- ❑ _____

Mood for Food

Canned food group
- ☐ Soups
- ☐ Fruits
- ☐ Vegetables
- ☐ _____

Fresh produce group
- ☐ Fruits
- ☐ Vegetables
- ☐ _____

Meat and alternates group
- ☐ Beef, pork, veal
- ☐ Chicken
- ☐ Deli meats
- ☐ Fish
- ☐ Peanut butter
- ☐ Cheese
- ☐ Eggs
- ☐ Dried beans and peas
- ☐ _____

Snack foods group
- ☐ Potato chips
- ☐ Nuts and seeds
- ☐ Chocolate
- ☐ Candy
- ☐ _____

Oils and condiments group
- ☐ Salad dressing
- ☐ Mayonnaise
- ☐ Butter, margarine
- ☐ Vegetable oils
- ☐ Dips
- ☐ _____

Sugars and Toppings Group
- ☐ White/brown sugar
- ☐ Honey
- ☐ Jams, jellies
- ☐ Syrups
- ☐ Whipped cream
- ☐ _____

Frozen Desserts Group
- ☐ Ice cream
- ☐ Frozen yogurt
- ☐ Fruit sorbets
- ☐ Sherbet
- ☐ _____

THE END OF OBESITY

Once you have identified your "problem food(s)," it is important to know in what context that particular food item poses a problem to you. Could it be that the consumption of these foods are a result of conditioned eating or emotional eating? Gaining a sense of awareness is key. Now that you've gained awareness of your problem food(s), you need to take action. Establishing an alternate plan to eating may be helpful to you. Table 5, the activity table, may help you think of alternate activities.

Awareness of your emotions, external cues, internal bodily physiological symptoms, problem foods, how to differentiate between a true hunger and a false hunger and how to deal appropriately with each type of hunger are all important steps in your quest for weight loss. Listening to our bodies is vital in helping us all realize "The End of Obesity."

Food is your friend. Know your friend well!

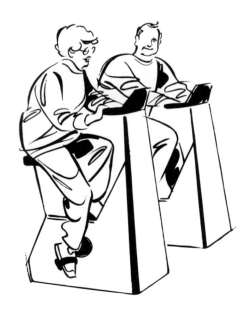

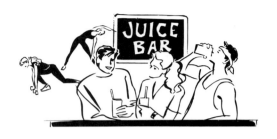

Chapter 10

At the Gym

"Use it or lose it!"
Anonymous

EVERY DAY YOU AND I SPEND anywhere from one minute to several hours fixing, cleaning, or maintaining one or more of our precious possessions. For example, think of the one possession that means more to us than we care to admit: our car. We wash and polish our car; we change its oil and rotate its tires; we even have it completely tuned up once in a while by an expert. Our cars are valuable to us. We need them to be available to us seven days a week, twenty-four hours a day. We depend on our cars to get us where we want to go. Admit it, we love our cars!

It's too bad that too many of us love our cars more than we love ourselves!

What have you done for your body lately? Have you given it a tune-up recently? Did you test-run it this week to see how it performs under demanding conditions? What kind of fuel are you feeding your body?

You depend on your body to get out of bed every day. Do you really expect your body to sit for hours at a work desk five days a week and then be able to perform at peak efficiency during weekend sports activities?

For maximum results your body needs regular use. We often say, "Use it or lose it" referring to people's loss of mental acuity during the aging process. The adage applies to our physical abilities as well.

You don't have to work out one or two hours at a time seven days a week to get your body running smoothly again. All it takes is twenty to thirty minutes of sustained enjoyment in the form of exercise at least three times a week.

Don't think you can sustain twenty to thirty minutes of intense exercise? Then break your exercise up into small and easily achievable portions. The end result will be a more productive, more energetic, and more youthful you!

Health experts agree that doing any exercise for even short periods of time is better than no exercise at all. You may not improve your cardiovascular system if all you do is ride your bike in a leisurely way along the local boulevard, but at least you will be burning some calories.

Why should you exercise? Why get your body to function better? Perhaps an analogy might help. Suppose you are the owner of a reliable and trusted car. Your car has never failed to get you to your appointed destination. Over the years you have dutifully brought it to the mechanic's garage for its required maintenance, including check-ups and oil changes. However, you have never spent a dime on fixing or replacing older or worn parts unless absolutely required. You dealt only with the bare essentials. The rest waited—and waited. Eventually, old parts of the car needed replacement: brakes, steering, radiator, transmission, fuel pump. You paid for the necessary repairs, all the while wondering why your car was letting you down more often.

At the Gym

Now, suppose you have the same car except that it's brand spanking new. You decide to bring your new car to the mechanic's garage a little more often for oil changes and preventive maintenance. You rotate your tires more frequently. The joints are greased regularly. On cold winter days, you plug the car's engine in to keep it warm. This last maneuver protects the engine from excessive wear and tear each time it is started in cold weather.

Five years pass and all is well. Ten years pass. The car that you would have had to replace by now due to aging parts and poor performance is still running smoothly. Fifteen years and half a million miles later, you give your well-maintained car to your teenage child.

Do you see the difference? The obvious point is that regular maintenance works not only for cars but also for the human body. If you maintain your body during its youth and on into early, middle, and late adulthood, it will continue to work better and longer for you and you will have much less chance of breaking down.

You do want to be around to share your accumulated wisdom with your children's children, don't you? You can—if you hang around. Just like the fifteen year-old car you pass on to your teenager, your wealth of experience can be yours to pass on to your descendants.

It's never too late to start taking better care of your body. Why not start today?

Once you learn to fly and can touch the sky, you will never settle for merely being able to walk on the ground. When you have felt the awesome power of good health and vitality through regular exercise and proper body maintenance, would you ever want to regress to a sedentary lifestyle that dooms you to a mediocre and mundane existence?

The End of Obesity

Fortunately, most Americans have learned of the benefits provided by regular exercise. Be sure to exercise with the proper basic equipment. Comfortable sneakers and a proper warm-up routine, including five to ten minutes of safe and slow muscle stretches and a similar cool-down period at the end of your exercise, will help you enjoy exercise as a lifelong activity with your family and friends.

The advantages of frequent and healthy physical activity are plentiful. Here are the most important advantages:

Cardiovascular fitness

There are two types of exercise: aerobic and anaerobic. Aerobic exercise, such as brisk walking, running, biking and more, increases your cardiovascular fitness. When you exercise aerobically you improve your body in two ways: 1) your lungs will be better able to extract oxygen from the air you breathe and 2) your heart will do a better job of delivering oxygen to the cells of your body.

Anaerobic exercise, on the other hand, such as situps, pushups and weightlifting, has no beneficial effect on the body's lungs or heart. Instead, this type of exercise usually targets the body's muscles and leads to increased muscle size and strength.

Aerobic exercise, if done three to four times per week for at least fifteen to twenty minutes and with the proper warm-up and cool-down periods, will dramatically result in improved cardiovascular (heart) health. The heart is a muscle. If it is exercised and made to work at a higher level often enough, it is almost certain to beat more efficiently, pump blood more vigorously, and beat at a slower rate.

Over the course of fifty years the savings add up: your healthy heart will have beaten 25 million times less then someone else's unfit heart and will be up to ten years younger than someone else's tired and out of shape heart. Ultimately, your heart will be less prone to the disease of modern living we know as coronary artery disease.

A Sense of Well Being

Most people who exercise on a regular basis feel healthier compared to when they were not as physically active. A runner's "high" has been well documented. It results from the body's natural brain hormones called endorphins (short for endogenous morphines) that are released during intense exercise. After a twenty-minute aerobic workout you will certainly feel better mentally. Ask anyone who exercises regularly.

Improved Oxygenation

Your body needs three things to exist: water, food, and oxygen. Your lungs deliver oxygen to your blood. Your heart then pumps this oxygen-rich blood to all of the body's parts.

As mentioned above, regular aerobic exercise increases the capacity of your lungs to take in oxygen from the air you breathe. This results in more oxygen delivered to the blood and, as a result, more oxygen to every cell in your body, including the parts that help you exercise: your arms and legs. More oxygen to your body parts allows for a longer and more satisfying workout before muscle fatigue sets in. The end result is more stamina and greater working capacity of your muscles, and less "huffing and puffing" by our lungs. Oxygen delivery to the brain is also enhanced. The net result may be an improved mental and intellectual capacity, allowing you to attain your top level of savvy and wisdom.

Improved Cholesterol

For more than a decade, cholesterol has been a hot topic. Most people think that cholesterol is just plain bad and should be avoided at any cost. Not so! In fact, cholesterol is a product of the human liver. The liver makes about 80 percent of the total circulating cholesterol in our blood.

What gives cholesterol a bad name is that it is one of the constituents of a blocked or "plugged up" artery. Blocked arteries cause most heart attacks and strokes. So, who in their right mind would think that there could be a good cholesterol?

Actually, there are both good and bad cholesterols. HDL (High Density Lipoprotein), referred to as good cholesterol, is a molecule that is made up of both fat and protein. This molecule is good because it removes cholesterol from our tissues and blood vessels, freeing our cardiovascular superhighway of potentially life-threatening traffic jams. HDL returns the cholesterol to the liver for recycling and elimination. The more HDL you have, the less cholesterol will be floating around in your arteries and the less chance you will have of suffering from a heart attack or stroke.

On the other hand, bad cholesterol, otherwise known as Low Density Lipoprotein (LDL), carries cholesterol to our tissues and arteries. A little LDL is needed because all of our body's cells depend upon cholesterol to maintain the structural integrity of their outer walls. Without cholesterol, our cells would lose control of their inner environment and die.

Too much LDL, however, leads to deposition of cholesterol onto susceptible areas within the body. Blood vessels subjected to both high pressure and high volume blood flow, such as arteries supplying major organs in the body (heart, brain, kidney, etc.), are the most likely to develop a buildup of cholesterol.

Continued accumulation of cholesterol may lead to "fatty plaques," the beginning of atherosclerosis, a term describing the hardening of arteries due to fatty deposition. Once atherosclerosis has developed, the next step may be partial or total obstruction of the affected artery and its consequences, which can be fatal.

But there is good news. Many athletes and regular exercisers show no evidence of fatty cholesterol deposits in their arteries. Why?

Apart from the fact that athletes are more likely to eat a properly balanced and nutritious diet, studies have clearly shown that regular exercise increases HDL, that good cholesterol (our hero!), the one you want in greatest quantities.

Just another incentive for you—if you are a reluctant couch potato—to get up off your soft and flabby sofa and run for your life!

Stress Reduction

Stress is a by-product of life in the late twentieth century. With the ever-increasing speed at which we live our daily lives, is it any wonder that stress has invaded our physical and mental well-being?

Just ask your local travel agent and you'll find out that tourism has become one of the world's top industries. However, you need not travel half way around the world to *run* away from your stress. Actually, that is the whole point. You *should* run, regularly, to help control your stress. You should bike, you should swim, you should play tennis, you should do whatever you enjoy doing to reduce stress and help your heart and lungs reach peak performance.

Exercise is a proven ally in the fight to reduce the stress levels of hundreds of millions of people around the world. Although there are other ways I could keep my stress level down without donning shorts and a T-shirt, I know of no better way to test my endurance and my stamina while purging my reservoir of stress than going for a run along the tree-lined streets of my local neighborhood. Try it! You'll see what I mean!

Weight Control

Weight control is the most important reason why Americans wear sweat suits or other exercise attire and pump their limbs and hearts until they are soaked in their own life-affirming perspiration. If it hasn't already been made clear, let me re-emphasize the point that exercise increases your body's operating efficiency.

Your ability to burn off calories increases if you exercise regularly. With a "souped-up" metabolic engine inside your body, weight loss is much more likely to occur. That muffin you ate for a snack will be burned off in no time when your body's engine is in high gear.

People who don't exercise will still burn off their calories, but at a much slower rate. The choice is yours: sluggish and idle metabolism without exercise or quick and efficient metabolism with exercise.

You would probably like to know the secret for achieving your weight goal—and maintaining it forever! Well, I'll let you in on a little secret: There is no one magic, foolproof way to lose weight and keep it off permanently. Nevertheless, with the right combination of a healthy lifestyle, avoiding dangerous substances such as drugs and cigarettes, wise food selections, and regular exercise, you can find your way to the promised land, where being overweight is but a distant memory.

The message is clear: America, let's get out there and put our bodies to work.

At the gym:

"Hi, Sophie. When did you get here?"

"About five minutes ago. I just started with my stepper machine routine, so I'll be another fifteen minutes. Why don't you hop onto the machine next to me?"

At the Gym

"OK. Why do you like the stepper machine so much, Sophie?"

"Well, I like being able to vary the pace of my steps easily to get either a light or a heavy workout. Right now, I'm at level 5. The easiest level is 1, and the hardest is 9. I'm doing the recurrent hill exercise program. Which program will you do?"

"I think I'll try the same level as you but on a flat and constant terrain. I don't want any surprises. Plus, I'm still trying to get the hang of this thing."

"Nothing to it, Sam. Just move your legs up and down, like when you are climbing stairs. Next, stand straight with your shoulders relaxed. That way you will be balanced and won't need to lean on the handrails like that struggling person over there.

"Proper stance is the key. You get the most benefit from your exercise if you use the equipment correctly."

"Same goes for all the pieces of gym equipment. So, how do I look?"

"Great, Sam. But you know, anyone can exercise just as effectively without the use of exercise machines."

"Yes. Running, walking, swimming, or playing tennis, for example."

"Right. I'll see you a little later on the track."

About fifteen minutes later:

"Wait up, Sophie! How come you're running today?"

"Sometimes I like to run. How about you?"

"I love running. I always have and always will. (See "Running With Dad" following this chapter.) Running helps me release my deepest thoughts and bring them to the surface. I've come up with all kinds of interesting ideas while running."

"Sounds good."

"Not only that. Running is a total body type of exercise. It involves the arms, legs, heart, and lungs. All involved body parts work as a team. The lungs extract the oxygen from the air and deliver it to the heart. Then, the heart vigorously pumps the oxygen-laden blood to the working arms and legs where muscles burn up the oxygen in order to propel the body forward. Don't you just love it?"

"Of course. Enjoy your run. I think I'll head on over to the weight room. See you soon."

Ten minutes later:

"Sam, wait up!"

"Are you already finished with the weights?"

"Yes, I am. Don't you want to take a break?"

"Sure. Let me just slow my running pace for a few minutes while I cool down. Then I need to stretch. I am so inflexible."

"Why is that?"

"I've been like that ever since I can remember. I've had to learn to stretch more effectively to compensate. I don't bounce anymore when stretching out my calf muscles, hamstrings, or quadriceps like I used to. I maintain my position for ten to fifteen seconds, then relax ever so slightly for another five seconds. I then stretch some more and hold that position for another ten to fifteen seconds, then ease off for five seconds before switching to the next muscle. In all, I stretch for about three to five minutes, depending on how tight my muscles feel.

"There are many benefits to stretching: prevention of muscle injury, improved overall flexibility, and an all-around enhanced workout."

"Do you stretch before, during, or after exercising?"

"I usually stretch before and after my workout. But I'm careful. Before working out, muscles are usually "cold" and tight. Stretching too rigorously may tear your muscles. Ideally, stretching should be done approxi-

At the Gym

mately ten minutes after you start your exercise regimen. By then the muscles have had time to loosen up so that they stretch easier. Stretching after a workout is also helpful. Your muscles can then tolerate a nice, long, relaxing stretch. Whatever routine you develop, stretching should be an important part of your exercise regime."

"How about that break now?"

In the snack room at the gym:

"Sophie, I am really hungry—and thirsty. What's the best food or drink that will give me the extra energy I need to power me through my workouts?"

"Before we discuss foods for fitness, we need to differentiate between short-duration and long-duration activity. Nutrition requirements depend on the type, duration, and intensity of the activity.

"Let's begin with short-duration activity. This activity lasts up to one hour. The majority of people are involved in this type of activity. Examples include a brisk walk or jog of twenty or thirty minutes, a tennis or volleyball game, an aerobics class, and the use of a treadmill or stepper at the gym. Most people engage in a short-term exercise a couple of times a week.

"To enhance your performance, here are some nutrition tips on what to eat and drink before, during, and after a short-duration activity:

"First, make sure you balance your meals using a variety of foods found in the Food Guide Pyramid. Ensuring adequate nutrition is key. Nutrients are easily supplied by a diet containing whole grains and cereals, fruits, vegetables, milk and dairy products, and meat, fish, and poultry. You also want to make sure you drink adequate fluids at each meal, especially prior to physical activity. Fluids can be in the form of water, unsweetened juice, herbal tea, or even a bowl of soup or bouillon. Alcoholic and caffeinated beverage choices prior to physical activity are not recommended since they increase fluid losses in the urine.

"During your workout, if you feel the need to drink something, your best choice is water. Following your short-duration exercise, it is always a good idea to help yourself to another glass of water, and keep drinking until you are comfortably replenished. Good snacking choices are also key for quick, pick-me-up energy boosters. I'll talk about them shortly.

"The second type of exercise is known as the long-duration activity. This type of activity lasts over an hour and includes marathon and endurance runs, long-distance swimming, and competitive athletics. Coaches encourage athletes to follow a diet high in complex carbohydrates and low in fat throughout the training period. Carbohydrate loading—eating a meal high in carbohydrates consisting of breads, cereals, rice and pasta—is a common occurrence during an athlete's pre-competition meal. This meal should be eaten two to four hours prior to the competitive event.

"Hydration is also important in maximizing the competitive athlete's performance. Eight to sixteen ounces of water are recommended one to two hours before exercising and another eight to sixteen ounces of water every hour during exercise.

"What about sports drinks?"

"The advertisements about sports drinks don't tell you the whole story. It is true that when you sweat you lose more than just water. Sodium and potassium also ooze out of your pores. The average weekend exerciser, however, does not need to replace those electrolytes immediately. Your usual diet will provide you with plenty of electrolytes, including all the sodium and any trace minerals that you lost from perspiration.

AT THE GYM

"Sports drinks, however, do have their place in the competitive athletic world where fluid replacement can make the difference between winning and losing.

"Water is still the best thirst-quencher and fluid replacement, and the best liquid to stave off dehydration and heat-exhaustion that we know. Speaking of which, I could sure use a drink."

"I'll go get us two bottles of water. What should I get for a snack? There are so many nutrient-rich snacks to choose from. My sweet tooth is tempting me to buy a chocolate bar."

"Fresh fruit or dried fruit such as raisins, apricots, figs, or dates are great energy boosters and can taste as sweet or sweeter than any chocolate bar you can buy. Since chocolate bars have significant fat, you'll actually be slowed down by eating a chocolate bar while your body tries to digest and process the fat."

"Wow! No more chocolate for me during my workouts. What about frozen yogurt, frozen juice pops or juice? Are they good snacks?"

"Yes, they are. These snacks supply a quick form of energy, so they are good choices for the individual who likes to snack between workouts."

"How about muffins?"

"As a general rule, muffins can be good snack choices. Be careful of muffins with a high-fat content. These muffins will slow you down."

"What about fruited or plain yogurt or milk? Are they good choices, too?"

"They're not ideal *during* your workout since they are dairy products. Milk and other dairy products are better choices *after* your workout."

"Why is that?"

"During a workout your body needs energy that is quickly absorbable and digestible. The natural sugars in fruit and juices are easily processed by our bodies within minutes. The protein found in milk and dairy products, however, take up to two hours for full digestion. Do drink milk and eat plenty of dairy products, but not in the middle of your vigorous exercise routine."

"Good point, Sophie. Switching topics: I've seen an abundance of ads touting energy bars and nutrition-filled candy bars. What's up with these healthy-sounding energy bars with 'everything' in them?"

"Without going into too much detail, why buy a Cadillac when all you need is a bicycle? These energy bars, which are geared more toward the competitive athlete, provide you with the same thing that fruits, juice, muffins, or other carbohydrate snacks contain: calories. The only difference is price. You pay more when you buy these bars but you end up getting virtually the same amount of nutrition." (See information below on energy bars.)

Energy Bars

Also known as sports bars or nutrition bars, these little bars are chock-full of what your body needs most during long-duration exercise: carbohydrates and calories. Carbohydrates are the best source of quick energy during a workout. There are two kinds of carbohydrates: simple and complex. Simple sugars include corn syrup, fructose, lactose, and sucrose, while complex sugars, also known as starches, include such foods as whole grains, rice, potatoes, corn, bread, and pasta.

An energy bar should provide at least half of its carbohydrates in the form of simple sugars. Anything less than this may decrease the central value of the bar's main purpose—quick energy!

Energy bars were introduced in the mid 1980s by Brian Maxwell of California. His personal quest was to find an energy supplement that could be eaten during strenuous exercise (such as running a marathon) and still be properly digested. His efforts resulted in the creation of the prototype energy bar: Power Bar™. Since this energy bar's successful debut, many other bars have

AT THE GYM

made their way onto the highly competitive energy bar market. We counted almost two dozen different types of energy bars on a local health food store's shelf.

Most of these bars contain between 160 and 280 calories, with the bulk of the calories from simple carbohydrates. The rest of these energy bars usually contain varying percentages of fat, protein, fiber, vitamins, and minerals.

Energy bars were designed and developed by a competitive athlete for the competitive athlete. Today, millions of non-athletic people consume them for three main reasons: convenience, taste, and the desire to feel athletic, even if only for the moment.

If you are looking for a quick energy boost that is relatively easy to carry, chew, and digest, the energy bar may be for you. Then again, so might a banana, a muffin, or any number of easily portable snacks. It's your choice!

"Got it, Sophie. I'll be right back."

Two minutes later. . .

"Here you go, Sophie. I got us bottled water and raisins. I also bought an apple and a banana. Which fruit would you like?"

"How about we share?"

"OK. They also had milkshakes at the refreshment counter. That reminded me of those flavored nutrition supplement drinks advertised for everyone from ages 18 to 99. What do you think of them?"

"These drinks will provide you with energy if you can't find the time to eat a sensible snack or meal. However, they contain mostly sugars and fats with small amounts of vitamins and minerals. This is because supplement drinks were originally geared towards people who were too ill to eat regular meals. Now they are being marketed to people from all walks of life."

"But what's the enjoyment of drinking a manufactured concoction? I'd rather bite into a sweet, red apple any day!"

"Good for you, Sam. Let's finish up here and get back to our workout."

"What do you feel like doing now, Sophie?"

Five minutes later. . .

"How about walking?"

"Sure! Did you know that some people think that walking is not a real exercise?"

"Oh yes it is. Walking involves all four limbs. Walking can also be tailored to your particular pace. Walking can be enjoyed after eating without interfering with digestion. You can walk after a meal and not get stomach cramps. Contrast this with running or swimming after a good-sized meal: your arm and leg muscles will compete for the blood flow with your stomach and intestines, resulting in inefficient digestion and possible stomach cramps. What's more, walking after eating leads to a fifteen percent rise in calorie expenditure!"

"I'm convinced. Let's walk. Do you remember when we walked sixteen miles (25 kilometers) up and down the hills of Montreal back in May of 1993?"

"Yes, I do. That's when you got the biggest blister I've ever seen!"

"I remember. I wore my oldest pair of sneakers. I learned something valuable that day: Invest in a good pair of sneakers for exercise. It costs much more later in aggravation not to buy a good pair of sneakers up front."

"I agree."

"While we're walking, I'm in the mood to talk."

"I'm listening."

"You may not know this, but in addition to prescribing medicines for my patients' ailments, I now prescribe exercise."

"You do?"

At the Gym

"Yes. For good reasons. As you know, the major cause of deaths in North America are related to an unhealthy lifestyle leading to heart disease, stroke, lung disease, diabetes, high blood pressure, obesity, and high cholesterol. These health problems are the cause for up to 70 percent of deaths in the US each year. The benefits of regular exercise are many: improved self-image, stress reduction, increased energy, overall sense of well-being, and more (see earlier in chapter). Additionally, exercise reinforces other positive lifestyle changes, such as healthier eating habits and smoking cessation."

"So how do you prescribe exercise to your patients?"

"I write it on my prescription pad just like all other prescriptions. However, instead of writing a drug's name, I write a description of an exercise regimen. With the patient's input, we determine the frequency, duration, and intensity of exercise, which is noted on the patient's prescription. For example, 'Walking 3x/week for 20 minutes at a medium-fast pace.' At each follow-up appointment, patients are asked to bring back their old exercise prescription in exchange for a new one."

"Do your patients actually 'fill' their prescription?"

"Most try. There is no shame in trying. I urge my patients to begin their exercise prescription by focusing on only one goal: to lace up their sneakers with their feet inside. Once a person's sneakers are laced up, the likelihood is much greater that some type of physical activity will follow."

"You don't push your patients that hard after all."

"On the contrary, Sophie. In addition to encouraging exercise, I also urge my patients to find ways during their busy day to do some form of muscle toning activity. Caught standing in line at the supermarket? Do leg lifts: lift your body by rising on your tiptoes with your right foot, repeat for a total of three times, then switch feet. Repeat. This is great for toning and strengthening the calf muscles of your legs. Waiting around for a friend or for a car ride? Put yourself to good use by doing arm exercises. Find yourself a wall, pole, or firm structure. Lean forward, use both of your hands, and push yourself until you are almost upright. Then lean forward again while still supporting yourself with your hands. Repeat for a total of ten times. Relax. Then repeat. In no time, you will have firmer and healthier looking arms. They may even be stronger!"

"Anyone can do these toning and strengthening activities almost any time!"

"Yes! And as the person's overall appearance improves, self-esteem increases, leading ultimately to stronger motivation to maintain a healthier outward and inward appearance."

"Sounds good, Sam."

"Thanks, Sophie. How about going for a little swim to finish for the day?"

"I'll race you to the pool!"

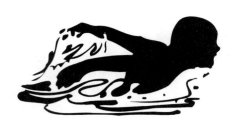

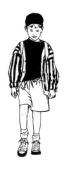

Running with Dad

by Samuel N. Grief, MD

A long, long time ago, during my carefree childhood, life was simple. I would wake up at 7 a.m., eat cereal with milk for breakfast, go to school, play outside with my friends, do my homework, then watch television. In between, mom would make my lunches and suppers and then both dad and mom would tuck me in at night, whispering "I love you" while kissing me on the forehead, the way parents always do. Life was so simple.

One childhood activity that I recall vividly—as if it were only yesterday—was going to one of the local high school athletic fields with my dad and running around the sports track.

For as long as I could remember dad had been an avid runner. For 18 years—ever since the day he and mom were married—dad had been waking up at the dawn's early rise to go for a run. Dad would wake up anywhere between 4:30 and 6:30 in the morning, depending on the season, put on his running attire, lace up his sneakers and slip out of the house without waking up a soul. One hour later, sometimes two, dad would quietly tiptoe back into the house through the garage door.

Before I was old enough to run with dad, he would run with a group of his friends each and every morning on the local mountain, known as Mount Royal. Their goal, as dad told me one hot and muggy summer day many years later, was to feel "as one" with the mountain. They would run through the woods, hear the crunch of fallen leaves underfoot, wake up the birds with their friendly chatter, and even meet the occasional novice runner experiencing the mountain for the first time. Thirty to 60 minutes later, after my dad and his fellow runners had completed their usual 5-10 mile circuit through the woods atop the mountain overlooking the city, they would then disperse, drive home in their separate cars and leave their running behind until the following day.

When dad finally thought that I was old enough to go running with him, we would go for a run around the block together when he got home from work. As I improved, dad began taking me to the local high school. Most of my running with dad took place on that high school sports track. The track was a quarter of a mile long (standard racing size) and was covered with slippery, sooty, crushed rocks. The first time I ran with dad on the sports track, I was only six years old. All I can remember was running a few steps, getting tired, and being picked up and carried by dad's big, strong and hairy arms. As the years passed, I learned to run with some style. My arms and legs, initially clumsy and inexperienced, eventually learned to move gracefully, pumping easily in tandem rhythm and cutting through the air aerodynamically just like dad's latest car.

Over the years, as my legs grew, I got better at keeping up with dad. At age 12, I was running with him, side by side, for up to two miles before I had had enough. Dad may have lost some running speed, but he sure was persistent. That was him in a nutshell: slow and steady.

It was during these runs that I learned why he enjoyed running so much. Sure, running outdoors delivered fresh air to your lungs while working off some of the day's stresses. Yet it was the strong, undeniably real, physical sensations that I felt while running with dad that made it so enjoyable and kept us coming back for more: the cool air entering my nostrils and flowing down the back of my throat and into my receptive lungs; the thud of my sneakered feet as they pounded the stone-covered track; the beating of my youthful heart inside my chest, quadrupling its regular workload to meet my body's increased demands; the occasional dull yet intense stomach ache I would suffer through, and ultimately conquer, as I pushed myself to run faster and longer; and lastly the sweat, salty and abundant, that oozed out of my pores, mainly from my face and forehead and trickled down into both sides of my mouth.

Dad's last running days were spent on Long Island, N.Y. during the summer of 1979. My two brothers and I had accompanied dad on this trip to see our American family yet again. Dad, as always, was up at the rooster's crowing hour, running along the empty streets of central Long Island. Five days into our summer trip, dad came down with a nasty cold and stopped his running until we got home three days later. Dad's cold symptoms improved except for a lingering, dry cough which stubbornly resisted a cure. Mom finally convinced him to see our family doctor. A physical exam, a chest X-ray, and four gruesome months of chemotherapy later, and dad was dead! He had succumbed to lung cancer, one of the deadliest cancers to afflict the human race.

Dad's running shoes collected dust.

In 1994 my wife and I packed our bags and moved south of the border to the U.S. There, we settled in New Hampshire, home of the "White Mountains." Not surprisingly, I have now developed the routine of going for a daily run. As I make my way through the mountain trails, stepping on dried up leaves and twigs and saying good morning to the singing birds of the forest, I sense my father's spirit. I imagine how he must have felt as he ran atop his favorite mountain. Even though I now forge my own trails, as long as I run I'll be running with dad.

The above article appeared in the September 11, 1995 edition of *Family Practice*.

THE END OF OBESITY

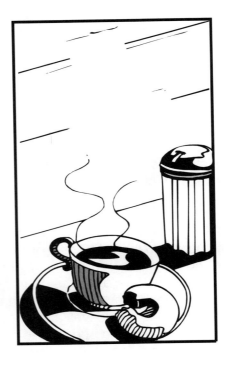

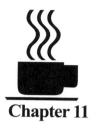

Chapter 11

At the Coffee Shop

"A really busy person never knows how much he weighs."
Ed Howe

COFFEE HAS EMBEDDED ITSELF into the heartbeat of the late twentieth century lifestyle. This lifestyle is at times chaotic and overwhelmingly busy, at other times sluggish and lazy, and often just a series of things to do one after another: places to go, people to see, tasks to complete. Coffee has infused itself into every aspect of our culture and filtered its way through all the pores of our society.

One might say that coffee is a way of life for many of us. Does the thought of not enjoying a refreshing cup of your favorite blend of coffee first thing in the morning put you into a panic? Do you become physically "discombobulated" when there is no more coffee in the kitchen and you have not had your daily "fix"? Do you go out of your way just to seek out your favorite coffee place in order to satisfy your cravings for the delectably deep and dark sensations of a cup of coffee?

You are not alone. Millions of North Americans, including most people in your community, are coffee drinkers. The search for a good—or better—cup of coffee is an ongoing "work in progress." As a relative newcomer to the coffee mania sweeping the world, I can see why coffee has created such a following. It's not just the coffee that has such an appeal; it's the settings and the accoutrements bestowed on your morning, afternoon or evening coffee that has such a dominating effect on your visual, olfactory, and gustatory senses.

Sophie was a regular coffee drinker when I first met her. I was not. Inexplicably, the addictive allure of coffee had not ensnared me through four years of medical school, several years of post-medical school studying, and three years of working as a family doctor in rural Canada. But, after marrying the woman of my dreams and moving to New England, I could no longer withstand the inevitable: I began to drink the most popular beverage of the world—coffee. Now that I am among the majority, I luxuriate in my addiction. However, my coffee habits are anything but ordinary. My addiction is not to coffee itself but to the **coffee shop**!

One of my most enjoyable leisure activities is meeting my wife at the local coffee shop. Indulging myself now and then with a cup of my favorite dark and deeply delicious brew, with or without a coffee shop snack, helps me keep my stress level hovering at its current low level. Of course, "coffee talk" relaxes me, too. Oh, there's Sophie now! "Hi, Sophie. I'm glad you could join me this afternoon."

"I enjoy our dates at this quaint little coffee shop. The coffee is superb!"

"I agree. Let's order."

A few minutes later:

"Sophie, I feel like talking about coffee and what goes into it. Specifically, I would like to know how healthy coffee is for me and if I should be concerned at all about enjoying my beverage."

AT THE COFFEE SHOP

"Sam, you already know the answer to that!"

"Tell me anyway."

"OK. You enjoy your cappuccino while I talk about caffeine for a minute. Caffeine is the most studied and best known component of coffee. It's the caffeine that gives all coffee drinkers their desired 'buzz.' The degree of increased mental alertness varies from individual to individual, but it is almost universal."

"Right. Excess caffeine, usually in the form of America's most popular beverage, coffee, will contribute to high blood pressure, heart palpitations, anxiety, nervousness, acid indigestion and frequent trips to the bathroom."

"Seems like caffeine is the issue here, not necessarily coffee. Sam, why don't I mention to our reader some of the other caffeing-containing beverages?"

"Go ahead, Sophie."

"Well, there are several. Cola drinks of all types and some other soda drinks contain a significant amount of coffee, unless they are decaffeinated. Decaffeinated beverages contain caffeine, but in minimal amounts. Other caffeinated beverages include most teas (except herbal teas), iced tea or iced coffee, chocolate milk, cocoa, and hot chocolate."

"What about caffeinated water beverages available at most grocery stores?"

"Yes, Sam. Those caffeine-filled water beverages are a recent addition to the types of caffeine drinks consumers may choose."

"The bottom line about caffeine in coffee or any other caffeinated beverage is to enjoy your caffeine in moderation—fewer than four cups a day—and you will be less likely to suffer any ill effects from caffeine."

"Caffeine is also found in other products like over-the-counter (OTC) pain relievers. Sam, should the reader be concerned about these pain relievers?"

"Good point, Sophie. Generally, OTC pain and headache relievers contain aspirin, acetaminophen, or ibuprofen. Caffeine is added to enhance the effectiveness of these pain relievers. The amount of caffeine in just two pain pills can equal the amount of caffeine found in a cup of regular coffee. Surprisingly, the OTC medicine you're using to treat your headache may contribute to 'rebound headaches' later on."

"Sam, can you elaborate for the reader about the link between caffeine and rebound headaches?"

"Of course. You see, for years caffeine has been known to relieve headaches of various types, especially the dreaded migraine. Drink one or two cups of strong coffee or other caffeinated beverage, and there is a good chance your headache may subside. There is a downside to this caffeine-headache connection, though. Once the caffeine leaves your system four to six hours later, your headache may return in full force. This is the phenomenon referred to as a 'rebound headache.'"

"How does caffeine actually help treat headaches?"

"Without getting too technical, I'll just explain that caffeine constricts blood vessels throughout the body, including the brain. Certain types of headaches occur when some of the brain's blood vessels dilate (open up) too much. Caffeine works by narrowing these excessively opened blood vessels, thus reducing the pounding or pulsations that accompany the headache. However, I wouldn't recommend drinking a caffeinated beverage for an evening or night-time headache or you might have trouble falling asleep!"

"Maybe if you drank a warm glass of milk—"

"—Speaking of milk. Sophie, let's talk briefly about milk and its fat content. The reader may be interested in knowing the differences between the various types of milk available to drink and to add to their coffee."

AT THE COFFEE SHOP

"First let's point out that milk contains many essential nutrients, including calcium, riboflavin, phosphorus, vitamins A and D, protein, and water. Most types of milk contain almost equal amounts of these nutrients. However, there is a noticeable difference in fat content. Whole milk is high in fat, a total of 3.25 percent fat by volume; an 8-ounce glass of whole milk contains 150 calories and 8 grams of fat. Two percent milk has a little less fat (5 grams) and provides you with 120 calories per glass. One percent milk has even less fat (2 grams), and one glass delivers 100 calories. Finally, skim milk contains little if any fat (up to 0.5 grams) and offers only 90 calories per glass."

"What about adding cream to coffee?"

"Cream packs a powerful punch of calories: about 30 to 40 calories per tablespoon."

"Sophie, what's your recommendation regarding milk or cream in coffee?"

"Ultimately, your goal is to choose milk with less fat in order to reduce the fat-related calories. So use a lower-fat milk in your coffee whenever possible."

"Sophie, all this talk about coffee and milk has revved up my appetite. How would you like something to eat? I'm getting myself a muffin."

"How about we share a muffin?"

"That's fine. Muffin coming right up."

A minute later...

"Here's our muffin, Sophie. Wow! It tastes very sweet and moist."

"Sam, many commercial muffins contain high levels of sugar and fat. This makes the muffin taste sweet and moist, but it adds many more calories."

"How can we lower the sugar and fat content in the muffins we eat?"

"One way to control the amount of sugar and fat in muffins, or any dessert, is to make them yourself. That way you have control over what ingredients go into your food.

"By the way, I have an announcement for anyone who may be wanting to cut back on the sugar or fat content of a favorite dessert. Evelyn Pytka, a friend of mine back in Montreal, published a book of desserts five years ago entitled *Almonds, Raisins, and Mostly Muffins*. This is a great book for anyone who loves to eat desserts and is looking for healthier ways to enjoy them."

"Weren't you the consulting dietitian for that book?"

"Yes, and I can tell you first-hand that these recipes are nutritionally sound. And the desserts taste great!"

"I'll drink my cappuccino to that!"

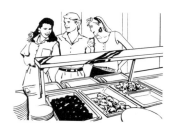

Chapter 12

At the Buffet

"When it comes to eating, you can sometimes help yourself more by helping yourself less."
Richard Armour

EVERY WEEK, MILLIONS OF Americans are invited out to some kind of festive affair. The list of potential social activities is familiar: a birthday party, an anniversary celebration, an engagement party, a wedding, a graduation event, a work-related festivity, a religious ceremony, a friendly get-together. What do all of these group events have in common? You guessed it. It's the method of serving the food and drink: the buffet.

The most popular way of offering party guests food and drink is by giving them full control over what and how much they can put on their plates. There are many advantages to buffet-style eating. First, as stated above, guests can exert total control over what they put on their plate. The second benefit is that the serving of the food is easy and orderly. Third, variety abounds on a buffet table, increasing the attractiveness of the food and increasing each guest's culinary experience. Another benefit is that the guest can go back for more of a favorite buffet item and, if one food item is not palatable, there are usually many alternative dishes from which to choose. Finally, because of the wide variety of dessert selections that are usually available, the last part of the meal is especially pleasurable. I am sure you can come up with more reasons why buffets contribute to a delightful dining experience.

Disadvantages of buffet-style eating do exist, however. Cold food may be warm and hot food cold. A favorite item may disappear far too early during the meal. There is always the potential for a bottleneck to develop at certain spots along the buffet table. Cutlery may be in short supply, creating a temporary inconvenience. If you become ill the following day it may be difficult to identify the culprit of food poisoning. Finally, and most important, the buffet plays to our all-too-human desire to eat, eat, and eat!

By now you are well aware of the alarming health trend affecting one third of adult Americans: OBESITY. Is buffet-style eating a contributing factor to obesity here in North America? Let's ask Sophie.

"Sophie! What are you doing?"

"I'm just doing the laundry, Sam."

"Let me take you away from all this laundry. I promise I'll finish up here later."

"Where are we going?"

"Into the living room. I want to sit down and talk."

"About what Sam?"

"Buffets."

"So—talk."

"I was wondering what you thought about them. Do you think they're good for people in general? Do you ever discuss buffet-style eating with your clients? Do you like buffets?"

"Whoa! One question at a time, please. First, I believe buffets have their place in our busy and modern

AT THE BUFFET

society. Buffets work well at big restaurants that cater to large crowds, especially on holidays and weekends. Buffets are fine when used for get-togethers and special events. Where else can you sample so many different and delicious food dishes at one meal? As a general rule, though, there is a lot of 'wastage' associated with buffets."

"Wastage?"

"Yes. The basic rule of a buffet meal is to keep hot foods hot and cold foods cold. Food poisoning due to an overabundance of disease-causing bacteria such as E. Coli can occur in susceptible foods that are not kept at the appropriate temperature. These foods include meat dishes, chicken, pork products, creamed dishes, and any dish containing dairy products.

"Cold foods such as salads, noodle dishes, and some desserts may also pose a health risk at the buffet table if they are stored and eaten as leftovers because germs may have been transferred unwittingly by guests from hand to utensil to buffet dish. To truly play it safe, all unused food from a buffet should be tossed out. That is why there is so much wastage!"

"OK. Any other comments on buffets?"

"Most people enjoy buffets for the variety of choices offered. People can select what looks appetizing and appealing to them. There's much less guessing and risk of a bad surprise or a disappointment than when you order a meal from a menu. At a buffet, your food choices are right before your eyes. There is one serious problem, though."

"What might that be?"

"A person with a particular food sensitivity or food allergy might find it difficult to know the exact contents of all the displayed food items at a buffet. If the buffet is catered, for example, it might be difficult to get an accurate description of some of the foods served. Although restaurant buffets might list the ingredients of each buffet dish, people with known food allergies should inquire with the restaurant's *maitre d'hote* or chef to find out whether a particular food item or specific ingredient was used in a desired food dish.

"Home-made dishes for buffets, on the other hand, are less risky as long as the person who prepared the dish is there to answer your questions. Ultimately, the safest rule of thumb I know is this: when in doubt, leave it out."

"I'm glad you brought up food allergies. Many of my patients suffer from food allergies. These patients should be aware of the potential for disaster at a buffet. Nuts, for example, are notorious for causing severe allergic reactions. They are often added to buffet-style dishes in small amounts to enhance the texture."

"That's right, Sam."

"One more thing I would like to discuss with you about buffets is the size of the plates available for people to use at the buffet. Remember, the underlying goal of our discussion here is to help the reader learn ways to eat healthier, lose excess weight, then stay lean. My personal feeling is that plate size is extremely important."

"No doubt about it. A hungry person given a plate twelve inches in diameter will almost always place more food on his plate than a person who is just as hungry but is given a plate only ten inches in diameter."

"Go on, Sophie."

"Most people fill their buffet plate to the point of overflow their first time through the line. All of us are occasionally guilty of putting too much food on our plates."

"I've been guilty of that many times."

"What better way to reduce the quantity of food eaten than by making smaller meal plates available for people? I'll illustrate my point with some basic math.

"Let's assume for our discussion that all plates are round. The area of a dinner plate with a 10-inch diameter can then be calculated using the following well-known equation:

At the Buffet

Area of a circle = πr^2
r = radius of a circle
and $\pi = 3.14$.
The radius of a 10-inch dinner plate is 5 inches.
Therefore:
Area of a 10-inch dinner plate = $\pi(5)^2$
 = 3.14 x (5 x 5)
 = 3.14 x 25
 = **78.50 square inches** of space available for food on your 10-inch plate

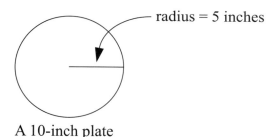

A 10-inch plate

Now, let's take a round plate with an 8-inch diameter. The radius of an 8-inch dinner plate is 4 inches.
Therefore:
Area of an 8-inch dinner plate = $\pi(4)^2$
 = 3.14 x (4 x 4)
 = 3.14 x 16
 = **50.24 square inches** of space available for food on your 8-inch plate.

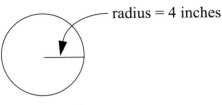

An 8-inch plate

As you can see, a two-inch reduction in plate diameter results in an approximate reduction in plate area of 33 percent!

Let's see what happens if the round plate has a 12-inch diameter.

The radius of a 12-inch dinner plate is 6 inches. Therefore:

Area of an 12-inch dinner plate = $\pi(6)^2$
    = 3.14 x (6 x 6)
    = 3.14 x 36
    = **113.04 square inches** of space available for food on your 12-inch plate

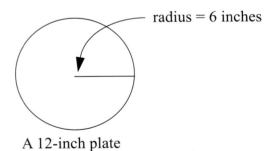

A 12-inch plate

"This time, a 20 percent increase i162

AT THE BUFFET

n plate diameter from 10 inches to 12 inches has led to an increase in plate area of over 30 percent!"

"Smaller plates mean smaller portions. This will lead to eating less. Right?"

"Not so fast, Sam. If we return to the buffet table for second, third, or even fourth helpings, then we are defeating the purpose of eating on a smaller plate. Also, making the right food selections from the buffet table is just as important as how much food you put on your plate. (For a more detailed discussion on choosing healthy foods, see Chapter 4, "Back to Basics: The Food Guide Pyramid.")

"What about beverages?"

"Careful beverage selection at the buffet table can help fill your stomach while providing you with fewer calories. Some of these lower-calorie beverages include carbonated or plain bottled water, unsweetened juices, an occasional diet soda, and sugar-free sodas.

"How about alcohol?"

"If you prefer an alcoholic beverage, keep it to a minimum. Even though alcohol may be part of the festivities, the calorie clout alcohol carries is impressive: Just one gram of alcohol provides 7 calories. Whether you consume a 12-ounce bottle of beer, a 5-ounce glass of wine, or a one and a half ounce glass of hard liquor or spirits, each of these alcohol-equivalent drinks will deliver anywhere from 95 to 150 calories. The amount of calories depends on the alcohol concentration of the drink, better known as its proof. The 'stronger' the drink, the more calories derived from alcohol. All of those calories, however, kind of take the fun out of alcohol."

"Let me get this straight, Sophie. At a buffet, you can fill your plate with good food, have a healthy beverage, and still satisfy your appetite without going overboard on calories.

"Eating slowly can also reduce the number of calories you eat at a buffet meal."

"That's right, Sam. As you know, the brain center responsible for telling you how full you are needs about twenty minutes to respond to the message from your stomach that you are full. If you are in a race to eat and shovel down as much food as possible as quickly as possible, you increase your chances of overeating and feeling uncomfortably satiated afterwards. The only way to stave off this overstuffed feeling is to eat slowly."

"It's too bad the brain doesn't get the message sooner that it's time to stop eating. I think the brain needs an updated fax or modem to speed up communication between itself and the stomach!"

"By the way, there is one other thing I'd like to talk about—dessert! Buffet desserts can be as varied as appetizers and entrees. The goal is to choose carefully. Indulgence during dessert is common. How many times have we heard people say, 'I'm being careful during my dinner to save room for dessert'?

"Often desserts are laid out on a separate table or readied for serving only after dinner is cleared. Regardless of when dessert is served, people invariably find room for dessert."

"Why do you think that is so, Sophie?"

"Because dessert offers a totally different array of taste sensations to a palate. It's like you're starting your meal all over again!"

"I see. With a new taste in your mouth, your appetite is rekindled. You are stimulated to pick up your fork and eat, regardless of how full you are!"

"That's how it works."

"What can we do to keep our calorie count down when eating at the buffet dessert table?"

"A **hunger scale** can help. By rating your hunger on a scale of 0 to 5 (0 means you are completely full, 2-3 means you are pleasantly hungry, and 5 means you are stark-raving vamished), you instill a sense of awareness and control of your food intake at the dessert table.

"At the dessert table, it is helpful to ask yourself: How hungry am I? If you are honest with yourself, you will know the answer."

"OK, Sophie. Say I am 1 out of 5 hungry. What do I do?"

"Go ahead and select your choices from the dessert table. Allow me to introduce at this time a corollary to the hunger scale. I call it the **out-of-ten rule**. The rule is as follows: eat only the number of bites from your dessert that corresponds to your level of hunger. To find out how many bites to have, multiply your level of hunger by two.

"For example, if you are 1 out of 5 hungry, this corresponds to 2 out of 10 and allows you to take a maximum of two bites from your dessert."*

"What if I like two desserts equally?"

"If you like, you can certainly sample more than one dessert, but try to stick to the out-of-ten rule. Ideally, if you are 1 out of 5 hungry, you will only take a total of two bites of your dessert, no matter how many desserts are on your plate."

"So, dessert is fine. Just enjoy enough of it to satisfy your residual hunger. Or, to adapt a famous expression: you can have your cake and eat a small piece of it, too. Thanks, Sophie. Let's go for a walk. I'll finish off the laundry later."

Buffet Blues

Mr. Thomas A., a single 56-year old man, came to see me (Dr. Sam) regarding his weight. He claimed he

---

* The idea behind this out-of-ten rule is to permit ourselves to enjoy a sweet temptation and not feel deprived ... or guilty. Deprivation eventually leads to excessive indulgence later on.

had always been in excellent health and currently had only one serious health-related problem: obesity.

His story was straightforward. My first question to Mr. A: Why do you think your weight is up? Mr. A proffered a knowing smile on his cherubic countenance as he admitted to me what had been going on for the last two years. As part of his new executive position at work, he was doing more traveling. Consequently, he was eating mostly at restaurants, either by himself or with his clients.

These dinners were often the all-you-can-eat buffet style menu plan, dessert included. Mr. A admitted that he had no will power when it came to food—especially at these buffets. He felt he had no control at the buffet table. Instead, it was the buffets that had control over him!

Another problem became apparent as our conversation progressed: Mr. A was not taking the time to take care of his most valuable asset—himself! His exercise routine ranged from sporadic at best to non-existent at worst.

Mr. A and I agreed that his lack of physical activity in combination with his excess food intake at the restaurant-buffet dinners were contributing to his weight problem. In fact, he told me he felt the solution to his "food problem" was to avoid restaurants. We agreed, however, that this was not realistic because his career depended on taking clients out to dinner on a regular basis.

We also discussed the importance of exercise for Mr. A. Exercise would help increase his metabolism so that his body would become more efficient at burning off calories. Mr. A agreed to start exercising by briskly walking three times a week for up to twenty minutes at a time. Mr. A managed to schedule a walking routine into his appointment book. It helped Mr. A to view his exercise slots as appointments.

AT THE BUFFET

I then sent Mr. A to see Sophie for a nutrition consultation.

"Hi, Sophie. Could you tell me how your nutrition consultations went with Mr. A?"

"I met with Mr. A for a total of three visits. After you initially saw him and helped him to refocus his attention on exercising, he was motivated to make positive changes in his diet. He knew that his business dinners both in town and on the road had not been selected with his good health in mind."

"What recommendations did you make?"

"I introduced Mr. A to the concept of *grazing* throughout the afternoon. This entailed cutting up a variety of veggies like green peppers, carrots, and celery, for example, and putting this colorful array of vegetables in a small plastic bag or container. Mr. A could then graze on this collection of vegetables any time.

"Mr. A was eager to go along with my suggestions to order a vegetable-based appetizer (light on the dressings and visible fats), or a vegetable type broth prior to all of his dinner meals when he dined out. That way, he would not be so famished for his main dish, and consequently would overeat less often at his dinner meal.

"Mr. A also learned how to be more selective in eating the foods on his dinner plate that tasted exceptionally good, not just average."

"What does that involve, Sophie?"

"I taught Mr. A a lesson that is key to controlling your food intake at buffets and reducing your calories whenever you eat out. That lesson is to visually rank each buffet item using the rating scale called the **Visual Appeal Scale**.

"For example, if the buffet table includes five meat items, four vegetable items, and six grain items, you would select the top two buffet items within each food group which you consider the most visually appealing.

The End of Obesity

"To illustrate the above point, let's take the grain group. The six choices at our hypothetical buffet table include potato wedges, mashed potatoes, french fries, a pasta dish, a rice dish, and a couscous dish. Mr. A selects his top two choices which are the most visually appealing to him and proceeds to help himself to a serving from his chosen dishes. He will use this approach for the rest of the food groups."

"It's always a good idea before you use the scale to walk over to the buffet table and make mental notes on food items and their food category: grain, meat or alternate, fruit, vegetable, or milk group. The above rating scale gives you a greater sense of awareness of which foods appeal to you most and which foods do not appeal to you at all.

"Too many people eat because the food is already on their plate. When we eat foods that are not truly 100 percent satisfying in terms of taste, flavor, and texture, we end up with a sense of disappointment and eventually guilt knowing we've consumed unwanted calories.

"You are simply prioritizing the foods you will be eating. If the food item doesn't appeal to you, don't eat it. If that first bite is not everything you expected it to be, leave the rest and find a food item which will completely satisfy you. This process gives you a tremendous boost of freedom from guilt associated with having eaten a food item which wasn't even satisfying to begin with."

"Interesting."

"Yes, it is. For Mr. A, this lesson reaped many positive benefits. First, he began to take note of each food item's visual appeal. He started noticing the color, the texture, luster, and presentation of all the different foods at the buffet table. He then used the visual appeal scale and selected the top two food items from each food group. Mr. A quickly became more aware of the foods he was eating.

At the Buffet

"Mr. A also learned to slow down at meal time. He was used to eating quickly and going back to the buffet table two, three, and sometimes four times. He was surprised to learn that it takes about twenty minutes for the brain to receive the message that you are no longer hungry.

"It was difficult for Mr. A to slow down his eating, but he eventually succeeded by taking more time to chew his food, by taking a fifteen-second break between bites, and by placing his cutlery on the table every few bites.

"These changes in Mr. A's routine allowed him to be more selective with his meal choices and more aware of what and how he was eating. When he did opt for the buffet meal, he chose the items for his plate with care, not haphazardly. Mr. A was able to prioritize which foods he truly wanted on his dinner plate. As it turned out, Mr. A had a penchant for broccoli, fish of all kinds, and eggplant. He really liked ratatouille!"

"I'm impressed!"

"Occasionally, Mr. A would order *a la carte* rather than dining from the buffet. Minor changes in his eating habits at the restaurant added further savings in calories for Mr. A. He began ordering his salad dressing on the side, dipping his fork into the dressing rather than pouring the entire cup of dressing onto his salad. He would request a bigger order of vegetables and a smaller portion of meat. He learned not to be shy about leaving some food on his plate or asking for a doggie bag. He would finish his meal with his choice of dessert in accordance with the out-of-ten rule.

"He realized that leaving a bite or two of his favorite food on his dinner plate would help instill a sense of control and power over his eating habits. He no longer needed to fear his visits to the restaurants or buffets, because he felt in control of his situation."

"Sophie, would you like an update on how he's doing?"

"Sure."

"At his last visit, Mr. A told me he had started up a swimming and walking program, every Monday, Wednesday, and Friday. The exercise has helped him relax and deal with stress more effectively. He is no longer apprehensive about eating at restaurants and buffets. Now he looks forward to going on his business trips, especially to try out new fitness facilities and the restaurant cuisine. All of these changes have resulted in Mr. A's having lost a total of thirty pounds over the last five months. He definitely is a healthier and happier man."

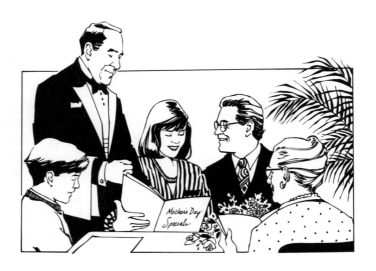

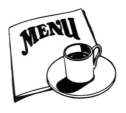

Chapter 13

At the Restaurant

"Food, glorious food..."
Charles Dickens, *Oliver*

EATING OUT IS ONE OF OUR FAVORITE collective activities. Americans eat out regularly. According to recent restaurant industry surveys, Americans eat more than twenty percent of their meals in restaurants, cafeterias, pizza parlors, "submarine" sandwich shops, and other fast-food restaurants. Fast-food establishments account for four out of every ten meals eaten out.

We eat out for many different reasons: business meetings, social events, to pass the time, as a leisure activity, while on vacations, or because we are just too busy or tired to prepare our meals at home. Eating out is a way of life in the late twentieth century.

Another important reason for the enormous popularity of eating out at restaurant establishments can be summed up in three little words: work, work, and work. Americans eat out during their work day on a routine basis. It has become a common office-site occurrence to see the office staff exiting promptly at their mid-day break to go to their favorite restaurant.

The End of Obesity

Americans are probably the most prolific restaurant eaters in the world. Drive along your local main street or shopping district. The vast selection of restaurants you see is outnumbered only by an even wider choice of stores and shopping malls. Sophie and I realize how much all of us have learned to look forward to or even depend on the restaurant as a source of food in our busy lives.

Americans love choice, and restaurant menus offer a bountiful selection of food and drink items from which to choose. At a restaurant or fast-food establishment, you can order any one of dozens of different varieties of hamburgers. And each of these hamburgers comes with a unique name along with a special array of toppings. Why have a plain hamburger at home when you can have the Big Mac™ with "two all-beef patties, special sauce, lettuce, onion, cheese, tomatoes, pickles, and mustard all on a sesame seed bun"? The list of restaurant names for hamburgers has grown since the Big Mac's introduction by Ray Croc almost forty years ago. Your own home-made hamburger has never faced stiffer competition.

What about all the other choices of cuisine that restaurants offer the hungry masses? You can choose from Italian, French, Greek, Chinese, Mexican, Japanese, Thai, Polynesian, German, or even kosher fare, plus the vast array of food offered by traditional American cuisine. It is a culinary jungle out there!

Come join in on the discussion between myself and Sophie as we visit one of our favorite restaurants.

It's pretty busy here. As usual, Sophie and I are seated in the far corner of the restaurant with a full view of all the action. Sophie's busy at the moment checking her messages. While we're waiting for her, let me share a little story about Sophie and myself.

We first met each other back in August, 1991. Five minutes after I met Sophie, I knew she was the one and only woman for me. The graceful display of her intelligence, accompanied by a large dollop of modesty, had me wistfully longing for our next encounter.

I soon learned that Sophie's demure outer appearance belied her secret passion for the pursuit of information on good nutrition and better health. Within two weeks of our first encounter, we went out on our first date. I took Sophie out to one of my favorite local eating establishments, where the food was always good—and plentiful.

After placing our orders, Sophie and I engaged in polite conversation. I learned that Sophie had just graduated from McGill University with a Bachelor of Science in Nutritional Sciences. She was a dietitian! And I had just ordered the eight ounce deluxe hamburger with all the trimmings, including French fries, cole slaw, and a root beer!

I squirmed in my seat as I wondered what she thought of my nutritional indiscretions. Let me tell you, I was extra careful that evening with my food. I chewed every bite of my hamburger thoroughly. Feeling self-conscious, I left half of it on my plate, not wanting to appear like my alter ego, the glutton, who had ordered my meal! Of course, I passed on dessert that evening.

A few months later, as Sophie and I were falling in love, I confessed to Sophie my embarrassment over our first shared restaurant meal. She smiled and said, "Sam, I love you for who you are, not for what you eat." Sweet words from the sweetest person I know. We all should follow her lead. Love yourself for who you are, not what you eat.

But, pay attention to what you eat because you are what you eat. Sounds simple enough. Here comes Sophie.

"Sam, what looks good on the menu?"

"Actually, everything looks great. I've been looking forward to coming here all week—especially so that we can have an intimate and relaxed dinner, with plenty of stimulating conversation."

"That's sweet. What would you like to talk about?"

"I was wondering why restaurants invariably offer a menu of foods that look scrumptious, taste delightful, but for the most part are overloaded with far too much of what all of us are trying to avoid."

"You must be referring to that biggest of little words: fat!"

"Exactly! And not just fat. Restaurants serve big portion sizes. The bigger the portion or serving size, the more fat—and calories—on your plate. Why is the public still willing to accept large portions at restaurants?"

"The only answer I can think of is because we, the consumers, want it this way."

"Why has the public not welcomed more low-fat or non-fat menu items into restaurants?"

"There is still a misunderstanding, perhaps even a fear, among the majority of consumers when it comes to low-fat or non-fat menu items. Some people have yet to fully grasp this concept. There also seems to be a stigma associated with a low-fat or non-fat menu item, a fear that it might not be as enjoyable as its "regular" counterpart. Let me share with you a story to explain what I mean."

"OK."

"Recently, during one of my busy work days, I took a friend out to a mid-day meal at a local restaurant. The restaurant was packed! My friend and I were lucky to get seated as quickly as we did. As we looked over the menu, my friend noticed a conspicuous absence of any low or non-fat items. For example, there were no 'lite lunch' or 'heart-healthy' items from which to choose. My friend was surprised and expressed disappointment."

"So what happened?"

AT THE RESTAURANT

"I told my friend that she need not be concerned. It is true that some restaurants have started to cater to the demands of the customers by offering lower fat and reduced calorie meals. However, the consumer should be aware that there are no set standardized guidelines as to what constitutes a low-fat, heart-healthy, or low-calorie meal at the restaurant. I explained to my friend that eating out the low-fat, low-calorie way involves more than just choosing food items from a low-fat menu. There are many other ways to reduce the fat and the calories when eating out at restaurants. (See below.)

1. To reduce portion size, order *a la carte* or share a large appetizer as the main course.
2. Request that dressings, gravies, and sauces be served on the side.
3. Order your meat, fish, or poultry broiled, baked, steamed, or poached rather than sauteed or deep-fried.
4. Be wary of foods that are "buttery," "creamed," "fried," "au gratin," or "marinated in oil" as these terms indicate higher fat content.
5. Have a spritzer (wine mixed with club soda) or a sparkling water with lemon or lime as your beverage to cut down on calories.
6. Relearn the art of leaving some food uneaten on your plate. Your body will thank you for it.

"You see, there are plenty of ways to enjoy your restaurant meal without all the unwanted fat or calories.

"My friend was eager to hear from the manager why none of the low-fat items she expected to see were on the menu.

"The manager came over. He was polite and pleasant. He explained that the restaurant owner (his first cousin) had recently labeled a whole section of the menu as low-fat. This was done in order to keep up-to-date with the ever-changing expectations of his clients. Surprisingly, the owner noticed a sharp decline in attendance shortly after changing his menu. It seemed that people were staying away in droves. Could it have been the low-fat menu section? Were people scared of low-fat restaurant meals? One month later, the owner got rid of the low-fat section in the menu, but secretly asked his chefs to continue preparing designated meals in accordance with his low-fat, low-calorie menu plan. Guess what happened?"

"People started coming back?"

"Exactly! The restaurant soon enjoyed the patronage of all of its regular customers again. However, now his customers were raving about his new meals—the low-fat ones that were not labeled as such. His restaurant has now become more popular than ever. What does this tell you, Sam?"

"That you can fool some of the people all of the time, but not all of the people—"

"—No, silly. I think it proves that even though Americans are more health-conscious than ever before, they have different expectations when it comes to low-fat meals. They still prefer traditionally higher fat meals because of their belief that it tastes better."

"Like I said, you can fool all of the people some of the time—"

"—Sam, give it up!"

"OK. I guess I'll try to order more low-fat, non-fat meals from now on."

"Sam, low- or non-fat menu items are not necessarily better for your health—or your waistline."

"They're not?"

"Take a look at the low-fat or non-fat dessert items available at restaurants, for example. Those desserts are usually quite tasty."

"Yes, they are. So what?"

At the Restaurant

"If a dessert item is short on fat it usually will contain a higher amount of sugar to compensate for taste. More sugar, more calories. Of course, now there are artificial sweeteners available to replace sugar and keep the calories down in our desserts."

"I prefer the natural taste of sugar. If I'm going to eat a dessert such as ice cream, I want it to taste just like I remember when I was a little boy. My father would drive my brothers and me ten miles just to go to our favorite ice cream parlor. It was worth it!"

"Sam, you can still have your high-fat and high-sugar ice cream. The problem you face is quantity. If you want your cake and ice cream to taste just like the good old days, you can enjoy them both. Just learn to enjoy them a little at a time. That way, you can have your cake *and* your ice cream."

"Sounds like you are borrowing my line: Eat less, enjoy more! But it may not be easy to stop after one or two bites of delicious cake or ice cream. How do I prevent myself from overindulging?"

"There are no miracle cures to help someone put down the fork. In addition to the out-of-ten rule mentioned in Chapter 12, you can maximize your dessert enjoyment by using the swish-then-swallow technique. Allow me to explain. Place that first morsel of delectable dessert in your mouth. As you do so, your taste buds immediately sense the sweetness emanating from the particular dessert. Once the sweetness is appreciated, each of us has trained our tongue to push the food to the back of our mouth and then down our throat where it quickly makes its way through our esophagus and into our stomach. The enjoyment of that food is over in a flash.

"A far better way to experience a dessert, and make the taste sensations last and last, is to swish the dessert around in your mouth so that your taste buds can fully appreciate the different flavors of that dessert.

"You see, our taste buds all belong to one of four groups: sweet, sour, salty, and bitter. Most of our sweet taste buds are located near the tip of the tongue, but some are also found on both sides of the tongue as well. The sour and bitter taste buds are grouped near the back of the tongue, a protective mechanism to help alert you not to swallow foods that have gone bad.

"To stretch out the sweet sensations that accompany the eating of a dessert, you can allow each bite to rest comfortably on the middle to front part of your tongue for a few seconds. This permits the sweet-sensing taste buds to fully appreciate their designated taste. Next, you then swish the dessert from side to side in your mouth. This swishing action helps to trigger the remaining sweet taste buds. The swishing of your dessert will actually prolong the sweet taste of your dessert, thereby satisfying you more. Besides that, you will probably not end up rushing through your dessert as most people do. This swish and swallow technique can help us learn to appreciate our taste sensations more fully, rather than our full stomach."

"That's like the wine experts during a wine tasting event. They swish the wine in their mouths and then either swallow or spit out the wine. They do this to maximize the wine's taste sensations. By the way, are you getting hungry yet?"

"Absolutely. Here comes our waiter. What will you have?"

"The garden salad with all those mixed greens sounds appetizing. Also, for my main meal I would like the grilled boneless chicken breast. How about you?"

"I'll be ordering the salmon, of course."

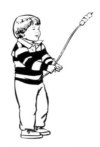

Chapter 14

Children and Obesity

"Children are our most valuable natural resource."
Herbert Hoover

HIGH BLOOD PRESSURE, DIABETES, coronary artery disease, high blood cholesterol, and obesity. These are medical conditions we associate with living the "easy" life provided by our relatively affluent North American society.

It's true! Our children are waging their own war against obesity, and in record numbers. Studies indicate that from 22 to 30 percent of American children are obese. Who would imagine that all of these seemingly adult medical problems could afflict our most precious possessions on this earth: our children?

Coronary artery disease, the condition in which fatty streaks and cholesterol-laden plaques build up along the lining of the heart's arteries resulting in a blocked artery and perhaps a fatal heart attack, is not just a middle-aged adult disease. Autopsies performed on American soldiers killed in action during the Vietnam and Korean wars showed that these young men, most between the ages of 18 and 22, were already well on their way to developing coronary artery disease. How come?

The answer is both as simple as can be and as complex as life itself. Our children follow us and learn from us. They mimic our ways. We are their role models. What have they been seeing us do for the last half of this century? Our standard of living has increased dramatically since World War II. With our technological advances, the need to forage for food or launch hunting expeditions for the necessities of life is a thing of the past.

Today we enjoy advanced communication tools such as the cellular telephone, television, computer, e-mail, and now the Internet, the most recently developed way of getting information to and from anywhere in the world. Why bother leaving the comfort of our home? Even if we leave home, private and public transportation are so readily available that we rarely walk, bike, or self-propel ourselves anywhere anymore.

Our lifestyle has become undeniably sedentary—and our children are watching!

On average, the American child watches between 20 and 25 hours of television per week. That's 20 to 25 hours of doing only one thing—sitting. While sitting passively for this length of time, it is easy to be influenced by the seductive, alluring, and mouth-watering television commercials for non-essential food items.

Children are trusting. They will truly believe that the commercial for a particular food product is 100 percent honest. After seeing a message dozens of times, a child will begin to crave a food product which promises everything to everyone.

Eating junk food and television are intimately related. As an intelligent reader, after thinking about the above, you might ask: Why do we allow commercials on television that are geared towards children, when these advertised products are not in the children's best interests? Answer: We live in a free and democratic society. The price we pay for this world-coveted liberty is freedom of speech for everyone, even if what is being said is obviously and blatantly hogwash.

Unless you have an electronic device attached to your television set that senses when a commercial is playing and blocks it out, the only realistic way to prevent your children from watching and listening to television commercials is to turn the television off. Period.

Children are children. With age and life experience comes maturity. You can use your own maturity to create an interesting physical and intellectual playground for your children. Ultimately, your children will be healthier, more curious about the outside world, and better prepared to face the future. Our children are our future. Let's help them to be their very best.

When I was a child, I briefly had a weight problem. I was born into a family with parents who grew up during the Great Depression or during the second World War. Families from those times were, on average, twice the size of the current American and Canadian family size of 2.1 children—and shrinking.

My parents knew hunger. They grew up on the poor side of town in pre- and post-war years. Their European immigrant parents had known only hardship in their home countries in eastern Europe and yearned for a better life. Opportunity for a better way of living and escape from possible persecution were the main reasons for my grandparents' migration to North America.

Visiting my grandparents was a regular event throughout my childhood. During those biweekly visits I witnessed the huge importance my grandparents placed on having an overabundance of food for everyone. Growing up as they did with daily uncertainty about their next meal, I could see why they were preoccupied with making sure that everyone was fed, and fed, and fed! Playtime was interspersed with delicious snacks or meals offered to me by my loving grandparents, during which time they would endlessly share with me their mantra to "eat, eat, eat your feet!"

This overt fascination with food displayed by my grandparents rubbed off to a certain extent on both of my parents as well as on me. No food could ever be left uneaten at the dinner table at my parents' house. My father and mother would start out by encouraging, then insisting, that I swallow every morsel of food on my plate. The most common reason used by my parents to get me to eat was their line about children starving in Biafra. I secretly wished that all the starving children could be given my leftovers!

That's how the habit of "cleaning my plate" developed. Even though I was not hungry anymore, I would still shovel whatever food remained on my dinner plate into my reluctant mouth. My stomach was the unwilling recipient of many meals to excess, and it eventually grew to accommodate the extra servings of food which I regularly delivered its way. I became a chubby child. Luckily for me, adolescence and the pubertal growth spurt cured me of my excess body fat. Not all children are so lucky.

"Sophie, I need some advice on how to manage a patient of mine."

"How can I help?"

"Timmy is a nine-year-old boy, the second of three children. Timmy likes to play video games, especially Nintendo, as well as play on the computer.

Children and Obesity

He's a very bright and witty boy. Unfortunately, he has a weight problem."

"How much of a weight problem?"

"Timmy weighs almost 140 pounds, and he's only 4 feet, 4 inches high. You might say that Timmy is really overweight."

"I think the term you are looking for is severe to morbidly obese."

"Why do we need to distinguish between the terms 'overweight' and 'obese'?"

"Obesity is an excess accumulation of body fat. In contrast, overweight can be either extra body fat or it might reflect a large skeletal structure or muscle mass, or both."

"I see. Anyway, his mother and father came with Timmy to my office recently to discuss Timmy's weight problem. I wasn't sure how to advise them."

"As you already know, childhood obesity is not an uncommon finding. In fact, obesity is the most common nutritional problem among children. The incidence of obesity in preschool age children is between 10 and 15 percent and increases to 30 percent in the adolescent age group."

"Not good news. By the way, both of Timmy's parents appeared to be obese, too. I felt a little uncomfortable explaining to them how it might be a good idea for them as well as Timmy to lose some weight. The parents are not my patients, and I did not want to offend them."

"It is a dilemma, Sam. But in reality, a family with obese parents often leads to a family with obese children. Both environment and heredity are important in the development of obesity. When both parents are obese there is up to an 80 percent chance that the children will become obese. When only one parent is obese the chance of a child becoming obese plummets to 14 percent."

"Too bad children can't all have lean and healthy parents."

"But remember, Sam, not all obese people choose to be obese. For example, certain disease states such as glandular disorders and genetic medical conditions, and certain medications all can contribute to obesity. However, for the majority of people, lifestyle is the main reason for their unhealthy weight."

"Right. Part of lifestyle is exercise. The only way to get a child interested in physical activity is to lead by example. Choose an activity the whole family would like to do together. Maybe your children would like to join you in ice skating, roller blading, swimming, or just plain walking. The important thing is to start relatively early in the child's life and build on success so that your child will want to continue exercising for the rest of his or her life."

"In reiterating your very important point about exercising as a top priority for children, it's important to understand that exercise also helps to conserve lean body mass, or muscle, while allowing for loss of fat.

"What this means is that you shouldn't drastically cut your child's total calorie intake. First, this may lead to loss of lean body mass and may cause delayed growth and problems with the central nervous system. Secondly, your child's body will adapt just as an adult's body will to the severe reduction in food intake by slowing down its metabolism. The end result is poor nutrition, an increased likelihood of developing vitamin and mineral deficiencies, and minimal loss of fat—and an unhealthy child!"

"OK. I'll advise Timmy's parents to encourage him to play outside whenever possible so that he's not sitting in front of the television or the computer playing video games. Seems easy enough. The way I see it, a parent's highest priority should always be the health and welfare of the child."

"I agree. By the way, did you get a chance to talk to Timmy's parents about what they feed him for his meals and snacks?"

"I asked them to identify some of Timmy's favorite foods. They said he likes cheeseburgers, chocolate chip cookies, and chocolate bars. Then Timmy himself added, 'And don't forget the banana splits!' What do you think Sophie?"

"The best way to make any headway with Timmy is to first educate the parents about basic nutrition. Your primary goal is to get Timmy to eat a healthy and balanced diet. But to do that, you may need to help modify the parents' eating habits as well."

"It is the parents who are in charge of buying and bringing home the food from the store. So long as the parents provide healthy food choices at home, both at meal and snack time, then at least the child will not be eating high-fat, low nutrition foods at home.

"It may be difficult to control what your child eats when away from home—at school, camp, or play. But, a little bit of the not-so-healthy foods such as potato chips, ice cream or candy bars won't hurt anyone if eaten once in a great while. Don't try to deprive your child of the occasional sweet or fatty snack, but do keep all the right stuff at home. Then your child will learn what's healthy and what's not."

"Do you think it is all right if parents take their child out for an ice cream sundae once in a while?"

"By all means. The principle is to keep healthy and nutritious foods on hand in your refrigerator or cupboard and leave the sweet or fatty food choices for the occasional outing."

"What should I say the next time I see Timmy and his parents and am asked how much he should weigh for his age? Do I just calculate the Body Mass Index (BMI)?"

"No, Sam. As I explained in the chapter, 'A Dietitian's Perspective,' BMI applies to adults aged 20 to 65 and is the 1990s version of assessing health risk associated with obesity. The best way to figure out the proper and healthy weight for a child is by using a standardized growth chart. Standardized growth charts have been developed to help doctors and parents determine whether a child's weight and height are following a normal growth pattern. To check on your child's weight in relation to height and age, ask your health care provider to show you your child's growth chart at your next office visit. "As a general rule, a child whose weight is on or above the 90th percentile for his or her age is considered obese. If we were to plot Timmy's weight in relation to his age on a growth chart, it would show that Timmy weighs above the 95th percentile for his age, indicating obesity. This means that Timmy weighs more than 95 percent of all other children in his age group."

"What about in relation to his height?"

"A standardized growth chart for children would show that Timmy weighs well beyond the 95th percentile for his height."

"How can I help Timmy lose weight?"

"The best approach to weight loss in children is the 'growing into your healthy weight range' philosophy. Ideally, an obese child should maintain his or her current weight while not gaining any more weight. Through improved eating habits and regular physical activity, an obese child will end up converting excess body fat into leaner body mass. The net weight gain over time will be minimal, but Timmy will have changed his body composition, and therefore his overall health."

"I like that idea a lot."

"I would also like to add a few points about the overall approach to healthy eating for children. They are basic but very important for the reader to know:

1. Providing enough calories and essential nutrients to ensure proper growth and development is the number one priority in the feeding of children. Quality is just as important as quantity when it comes to making food choices for your child. A proper balance in food choices, based on the Food Guide Pyramid, will help your child to reach his or her highest potential, physically and intellectually.

2. Childhood is an important period for establishing healthy eating habits. What you learn in childhood usually stays with you for life. (See our discussion of parental role modeling earlier in chapter).

3. It is important for the whole family to establish an eating pattern that takes into consideration each member's specific needs while emphasizing variety, moderation, and a balance of grains, fruits, vegetables, meat and alternate protein sources, and milk and dairy products. Regardless of age, if all members of the same family approach their meal and snack times with a healthy attitude, healthy food choices will generally follow."

"Sophie, you mentioned that we should all eat foods from the grain group, such as bread, pasta and rice. Timmy's parents complained that he ate a lot of bread. They said they thought that eating too much bread was contributing to his current weight problem. What do you think?"

"It's a myth that bread, pasta, rice, and other grain products are fattening. These are among the very foods dietitians recommend for healthy eating. Grain products are excellent sources of complex carbohydrates and are naturally low in fat—unless of course, they are topped with a thick layer of butter, margarine, or mayonnaise or served with rich and creamy sauces."*

"OK. Should I counsel Timmy about eating a healthy breakfast?"

"Breakfast is the most important meal of the day for everyone. Eating breakfast helps kick-start your metabolic flame. Without breakfast, your body turns to burning left-over sugars or fats from last night's meal, but it does so in an inefficient manner. The result is that your brain does not get the right mixture of fuel it needs to perform at its peak function and you end up not feeling your best.

"You might think that breakast skippers can get all the nutrients they missed by making up for it at other meals later that day. On the contrary, studies have shown that breakfast skippers actually take in much lower amounts of several key nutrients than do their breakfast-eating counterparts.

"In addition, the overall dietary practices and diet quality of breakfast-skippers are not as good as they are for those who eat breakfast regularly. Chil-

---

* In reality, there is no one food that is "fattening." Some foods have more calories than others, but given enough time, calories from any one food that is eaten will be burned off. Even the calories from a chocolate bar will be used up for energy by the body and not stored as fat if it is the only source of energy available. It's the total diet over a period of time that determines weight gain and not any one particular food.

dren who skip breakfast have a decreased attention span compared to their breakfast-fed schoolmates. Ironically, consumer research has shown that many parents still believe that breakfast is not the most important meal of the day. Parents may transfer such attitudes and practices to their children."

"So breakfast should definitely be a top priority for Timmy."

"Exactly."

"Sophie, what is your idea of a complete breakfast?"

"A complete and balanced breakfast should contain foods from at least three different food groups. The typical breakfast most people think of consists of toast or cereal, milk, and fruit or juice. This breakfast meets the standard of having at least three different food groups: toast or cereal (grain group), milk (milk and dairy group), and fruit or juice (fruit group). During a rushed morning, here are some suggestions parents can use to improve the chances of their child eating breakfast:

1. First things first. Parents should encourage their children to eat breakfast by setting an example with their own breakfast habits. Mom and dad, eat your breakfast!

2. When working parents leave for work before children are up, easy-to-prepare foods can be left for children along with simple instructions.

3. When time is really limited and children refuse to eat breakfast, extra food can be packed along with lunch so that breakfast can be eaten in the car on the way to school or just before classes begin.

4. Planning ahead the night before can also be very helpful. For example, pour your child's favorite breakfast cereal into a bowl and wrap it appropriately. Then place cutlery and a glass along with the wrapped cereal bowl on the kitchen table. All that is left to do is pour the milk and juice in the morning."

"Sophie, I'm starting to feel more at ease about discussing obesity with parents and their children. But practically speaking, I would need to be able to recommend specific foods or snacks for children to eat. Same goes for breakfast. Do you have any ideas?"

"Yes, I do. The parents' hope that their child will have a hearty appetite and eat nutritiously is not enough to help a child achieve good nutrition. It is the parents' **attitude** toward towards food that establishes the pattern of eating at home for the child. If the parents are always in a rush in the kitchen and eat hurriedly, you can bet this child will be a fast eater, too.

"Examples of other actions that do not promote positive eating habits: Do the parents insist that the child finish off every last piece of food on their plate? Do the parents involve the child in the selection and preparation of some favorite family foods? Do the parents encourage, rather than discourage, their child's natural creativity with food?

"We need to see food from a child's perspective. We were all children at one time in our lives. Remember what it felt like to savor the crunchiness of a nut or an apple, the frosty creaminess of a cold milkshake, or the natural sweetness of an orange? The goal of parents should be to help sharpen their children's taste buds in order to appreciate the entire spectrum of aromas, flavors, and textures that different foods offer. The best way to do that is to have children sample a wide variety of foods.

"It is sad that because some parents give up so easily in showing their children the many benefits of choosing new foods, their children are left with a limited knowledge of foods—a clear disadvantage. They may never learn to savor and enjoy certain foods and the accompanying sensations that are not only wonderful, but good for you, too."

"It sounds like it's up to parents to help children learn about food. We can't expect our children to learn about everything in school."

"Right. Home economics is not enough. Besides, it's never too early for parents to involve their son or daughter in the planning, buying, cleaning, and preparing of food.

"It is never too late to foster a healthy interest and approach to food. Snacks are actually a good thing. Snacking between meals provides energy and nutrition that children's bodies need during a busy and active day.

"The kind of snack you and your child prepare is limited only by your imagination. Don't be surprised if your child comes up with a new and innovative snack all by himself. Don't just give your child milk and cookies for a snack, give him what he wants: variety."

Following are some snack ideas geared toward children **of all ages**, including adults!

Sophie and Sam's Fundamentals of Snacking

1. To eat is human, to snack is divine.

    Snacking for some people contributes a substantial portion of their daily food intake. Some people never sit down to eat their meals. They are constantly on the move, eating on the run, and have little time for a relaxing and satisfying meal. Snacks are the backbone of their existence. Living on snacks doesn't need to be a risky business. Choose foods for your snacks that are packed with nutrition.

    Try a bowl of fresh fruit consisting of grapes, blueberries, bananas, strawberries, or pineapple. Top it off with your favorite non-fat yogurt and a dash of cinnamon.

    Crunch on some fresh veggies with your favorite homemade dip.

    Pop your own popcorn and save calories by air-popping it.

    Breakfast isn't the only time to enjoy unsweetened cereal with low-fat milk. Sprinkle your cereal with dried fruits, nuts or seeds for added nutrition.

    Make your own muffins and biscuits to control the amount of sugar and fat that go into these snacks.

    For a homemade milkshake, mix your choice of fruit with milk or yogurt in a blender. For more volume, add a few ice cubes.

2. You can eat snacks day or night.

    No longer is working from nine to five the norm. People are working flexible schedules. Fewer people are eating at traditional mealtimes. Snacks can be invaluable in helping you stay healthy while working longer hours, irregular hours or the night shift.

3. **Bring on the snack attack.**

   Hunger pangs often strike without warning. These well-known stomach spasms can be the scourge of a busy day. Or you can welcome them for what they are: the sign of a healthy appetite and an efficient internal metabolic furnace. Take time to satisfy your stomach's request for food and help curb your body's energy cravings. This will lead to much less excessive eating at mealtimes. Not all hungers are the same (See Chapter 9, "Mood for Food.") Face up to your true hunger when it presents itself. Feed your body what it needs: healthy and wholesome foods from the five food groups. You'll thank yourself!

4. **Make SNACKs fun.**

   S = Size down. Make snacks small enough to be portable. That way you can take your snack anywhere.

   N = No need to prepare. Fruits and vegetables are tasty, simple, and require little or no preparation. Peel an orange ahead of time and carry it to work in a plastic container. Or bring a crunchy green pepper cut up into bite-size pieces. Make your own "office trail mix" with one cup each of sesame sticks, almonds and raisins mixed into a bowl. Come up with your own snack ideas.

   A = Aim for nutrition.

   C = Create and invent. Think of healthy snacks you'll want to eat every day. Use your imagination.

   K = King or queen, snacks are for everyone.

   So let's get snacking!

The End of Obesity

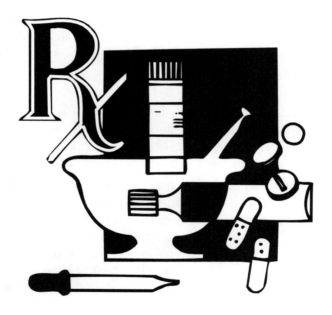

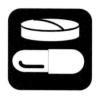

Chapter 15

"Magic" Pills

"I want a new drug, one that does what it should, one that won't make me feel too bad, one that won't make me feel too good..."

Huey Lewis and the News, Sports, 1983

BY NOW, YOU ARE PROBABLY aware of our lack of enthusiasm for all quick-fix approaches to obesity. Most Americans tend to gain weight gradually over the years. The pounds accumulate in our hips, our soft and cushiony bottoms, our legs and arms, and for most men, our stomachs, also known as "the pot belly." (See the following chart.)

Percentage of American Men and Women Who Are Overweight, by Age Group (1991)

Age Group	Men (%)	Women (%)
20-29	20.2	20.2
30-39	27.4	34.3
40-49	37.0	37.6
50-59	42.1	52.0
60-69	42.2	42.5
70-79	35.9	37.2
Over 80	18.0	26.2

Above chart courtesy of Wyeth-Ayerst Laboratories, Philadelphia, PA. Overweight is defined by Wyeth-Ayerst as being 20 percent or more above one's healthy weight range.

If there is a simpler, quicker, or easier way to do something, someone will eventually think of it, develop it, and try to sell others on their idea or product. Not surprisingly, the diet pill and diet product market is booming. Since the introduction of amphetamines (known in the drug world as "speed") and their over-the-counter cousins such as Dexatrim™—diet pills, powders, and potions have been welcomed by dieters as their best friends.

Marketers of these "magic pills" and related products tout the way they increase your body's fat burning capacity, decrease your appetite, build up muscle mass, lift your self-esteem, and help you become a successful person. No wonder these pills are so wildly popular!

Diet pills are *not* harmless. Common side effects of diet pills include dry mouth, sleep disturbance ranging from insomnia to excessive drowsiness, dizziness, abdominal pain, bowel changes, nausea, fatigue, and nervousness.

Many of these diet pills act on the brain and spinal cord of the central nervous system, inducing a more aroused state of awareness. Unfortunately, this increased level of arousal can prevent relaxation at bedtime. Consequently, most diet pills cause a certain amount of insomnia, a price to be paid for taking one or more diet pills prior to supper. Excessive use and abuse of diet pills can lead to palpitations, blurry vision, chest pain, seizures, coma, and even death!

As with many drugs, tolerance to most diet pills usually develops within a few weeks. That means you need to take a larger amount of the active ingredient in the diet pill for it to continue to work in decreasing your appetite. Unfortunately, side effects such as irritability or nervousness also increase as the dosage of the diet pill increases.

A popular medication for controlling the appetite is Phenylpropanolamine. Available in a wide variety of over-the-counter weight loss pills (such as Dexatrim™), this chemical has been used by millions of people seeking happiness through weight loss. Often, phenylpropanolamine is combined with caffeine in a single pill to raise the pill taker's metabolism, thus enhancing weight loss. People with high blood pressure or heart disease should be closely monitored and under the supervision of a medical professional when taking this medication. The daily dosage should not exceed 75 mg per day. Remember, you must weigh the benefits and the risks of taking diet pills before you begin. Check with your trusted health care professional.

The following drugs are available only by prescription:

Diethypropion (Tenuate) is a drug similar to amphetamines, but it carries much less risk to people with high blood pressure. It works just like amphetamines, by curbing appetite and stimulating the central nervous system. Side effects tend to be less severe compared to amphetamines. The usual dose is 25 mg three times a day.

Fenfluramine (Pondimin) generally causes drowsiness and is a preferred drug for individuals who are anxious and in whom overstimulation of the central nervous system should be avoided, such as people with epilepsy. Fenfluramine should not be given to patients who are depressed, on antidepressants, or who are taking other drugs with similar central nervous system effects. The usual dosage is 20 to 40 mg three times a day. Recently, this medication has been taken off the weight-loss pill market. (See "Redux Update" at the end of this chapter for the latest information on the safety of these diet pills.)

Phentermine (Phentrol, Ionamin) has become more popular in recent years since being introduced as a weight-loss partner to fenfluramine. Phentermine is a stimulant drug, thus increasing the body's metabolism. Its side effects are more pronounced than other prescription weight-loss pills, the most common ones being insomnia, nervousness, and dry mouth. The usual dose is 15 to 30 mg taken once daily.

Fen-Phen (fenfluramine and phentermine) was a popular diet pill duo in helping people to lose their excess weight and in keeping it off—until the government's withdrawal of fenfluramine from the market. Fenfluramine and phentermine are amphetamine-like drugs, but they have somewhat different actions. Fenfluramine inhibits the uptake and subsequent breakdown of a brain neurotransmitter called serotonin. Serotonin is well known for its involvement in relation to mood, sleep and arousal, and hunger/satiety. The resulting increased serotonin levels lead to a decreased appetite.

Other drugs that inhibit the uptake or re-uptake of serotonin in different areas inside the brain such as **Prozac** and other similar anti-depressant drugs have also been tried in the treatment of weight loss. The results have not been consistent. Studies have demonstrated only a limited amount of success in curbing appetite.

Phentermine, on the other hand, inhibits uptake of norepinephrine within the brain. Norepinephrine is an important chemical messenger used in the brain as well as throughout the rest of the body. The prevention of norepinephrine from being taken up by brain receptors leads to an increased overall basal metabolic rate, thus increasing the body's energy burning capacity. Taken together, the differing mechanisms of action of fenfluramine and phentermine resulted in more efficient weight loss for many people.

I would like to present the following story that took place from June 1996 to July 1997 of how fen-phen was prescribed for one of my patients in her quest for weight loss. The story is a real one, with some modifications. The frenzy of taking fen-phen and other diet pills has become prevalent in our society today.

Fen-Phen Frenzy

Miss C, 34 years old, was my last appointment on a busy Friday afternoon. She wanted to discuss her painful right heel. And, oh, by the way, she mentioned to me her desire to lose weight and if I could recommend anything for weight loss.

Miss C stood 5 feet, 3 inches tall and weighed in at 300 pounds even. She was morbidly obese. As our discussion progressed, I learned that Miss C had tried "all of the diets and diet plans out there," although she had never taken any over the counter diet pills nor had she ever been prescribed a weight-loss pill.

Deferring the weight issue for the moment, I examined Miss C's right foot and heel. After an X-ray of her right heel showed the presence of a bony heel spur, I prescribed an aspirin-like medication for her pain and suggested a pair of shoe inserts. She requested a follow-up appointment the next week to discuss her weight management problem.

One week later, Miss C came back to see me. Her heel now on the mend, she appeared eager to make a new start in regards to her weight. She shared her plans with me: no more late night snacks, no more polishing off a whole pie at one sitting, no more feeling sorry for herself and eating that much more in an attempt to console herself.

Miss C told me she had always followed short-term, very low-calorie diets in the past. She admitted that she always regained all the weight lost during her brief and intense diets, often adding on many more pounds in the process. Miss C said she wanted to take a weight-loss pill. I reminded her that a change in lifestyle was the key to unlocking the successful path to weight loss. That is, a combination of a liberal and diverse exercise strategy combined with healthful and enjoyable food choices, would help in achieving her weight-loss goals.

I referred her to Sophie for nutritional counseling with a special emphasis on behavior modification. Finally, I prescribed Miss C the diet pill combination: Fenfluramine and Phentermine (Fen-Phen). I explained in detail the possible side effects of these medications. (Please be aware that Fenfluramine and its new cousin Dexfenfluramine (Redux) have been withdrawn from the market and are currently considered unsafe for public use. See the section at the end of this chapter.)

One month later, Miss C was back to see me. She had made many changes in her lifestyle and in the way she was eating. She was no longer using food to fill the empty moments of her life. She had also learned to enjoy exercising. Her exercise program included a daily thirty-minute walk, a fifteen-minute swim every other day, and a weekly muscle training session with a qualified fitness trainer.

After six months, I told Miss C that I was no longer comfortable prescribing her Fen-Phen, as most of the human studies with this weight-loss pill combination had not gone beyond six months. She agreed to stop the Fen-Phen.

Here is the amazing part of the story. Miss C continued to lose weight at the same rate as she did when on Fen-Phen! Within nine months she had lost a total of sixty pounds. And in twelve months, a full year after beginning her new way of life, Miss C weighed just under 225 pounds. She looked noticeably leaner and felt much better.

"Sophie, what was your experience with Miss C?"

"Miss C was extremely motivated to lose her excess weight. Seeing that she was an emotional eater, I helped her to better understand her emotional triggers for eating. She made remarkable gains in assessing her hunger level and coping with her occasional food cravings.

"Other lessons Miss C learned included portion control, how to deal with 'snack attacks,' and cooking the low-fat way. Best of all, her self-image improved dramatically and she discovered the concept of giving herself permission to eat certain foods without the accompanying guilt that had been literally weighing her down. She also appeared intent on ridding herself of the heel spur on her foot. How has her foot been doing, Sam?"

"The last I heard from Miss C, her heel was not causing her any more grief! Seriously, Sophie, what do you think of Miss C's continuing to lose weight after stopping the use of Fen-Phen?"

"I'm not surprised, Sam. Miss C made realistic lifestyle changes and learned to make friends with food. She has come a long way!"

These days it is next to impossible not to come across herbal and other alternative diet pills in health food stores, pharmacies, even supermarkets. I believe it is fair to say that the modern North American doctor is missing the boat if he or she is not asking patients whether they are using herbal/homeopathic/alternative substances. The proliferation of these products is no accident. People are looking for the "miracle" cure. Instantaneous results are promised by the manufacturers of most of these "fat burners." And the advertising is working!

Non-traditional/alternative medicine has increased in popularity over the past several years and is now a multibillion-dollar industry. Naturopathy, homeopathy, chronotherapy, and many more alternative medicine disciplines are fast becoming part of mainstream medicine in our culture.

Dietary supplements comprise a large portion of this expanding component of our economy. The most common dietary supplements include herbal products like garlic, ginseng, gingko biloba, evening primrose oil, as well as multivitamins and mineral combinations, vitamin E megadose, vitamin C megadose, calcium, and more.

Alternative weight loss pills are also being gobbled up by millions of Americans as they desperately seek their elusive "perfect weight." Such weight-loss products include chromium picolinate (a mineral needed in minute amounts for good health), chitosan (a sea-food fiber extract), green-tea extract, garcinia, L-carnitine, and more.

The advertisements for these pills promise us what most of us would love to hear. Catch phrases with quick and easy one-liners fill the pages of magazines: "lose weight fast," "watch fat melt away," "no more dieting,"

"MAGIC" PILLS

"forget about counting calories," "lose weight 24 hours a day," "stop your body from storing fat" and many more.

Some of these products are potentially harmful, and their manufacturers claim that they are derived from rare plants, trees, or herbs located in far-away places in South Asia or in a tropical rain forest. A recent scare occurred concerning the herbal product "ma huang," also known by its more common pharmaceutical name of "ephedra" or "ephedrine." This product is a drug that can speed up your heart rate, increase your metabolism, and, if taken to excess may lead to seizures, heart attacks, and even death.

"Herbal Fen-Phen," a combination of two herbal products—St. John's Wort, a flowering plant; and ephedra, an ancient Chinese herb (see above)—has made its way into people's homes.

Whatever you call these alternative diet pills, remember that they are not subject to the scrutiny of the Food and Drug Administration (FDA) and can be easily obtained and used indiscriminately.

Just because a product is described as "natural" does not mean that it is safe for human consumption. Please ask your doctor or health care practitioner about all diet pills before you try them.

For every diet pill you have ever swallowed, think of all the missed opportunities that you had to enjoy a wholesome, nutrient-rich fresh food item. No diet pill can ever make good on the promise to bring you long-lasting good health. Only proper living, wise food selections, and lots of exercise can help you to accomplish your goal of good health.

Because of the widespread reporting among physicians regarding the health problems encountered by taking fenfluramine and dexfenfluramine (Redux), I have included a section in this chapter on Redux, the newest FDA-approved diet pill, which has recently been withdrawn from the market. The developments referred to in the following section came to light just prior to this book's printing.

Redux: background information

Redux, a drug that had been available in Europe for over a decade, was approved for public use in the US on April 29, 1996. The drug's chemical name sounds scary: (S)-N-ethyl-alpha-methyl-3-(trifluoromethyl) benzeneethanamine hydrochloride. Its generic drug name was dexfenfluramine, but North Americans knew it by its trade name, Redux.

Formulated by the research division of Servier of France, Redux was the first weight-loss drug allowed onto the prescription drug market by the Food and Drug Administration (FDA) in more than twenty years. Combined with a reduced-calorie menu plan, Redux was shown to result in both weight loss and maintenance of that weight loss.

Redux is a chemical cousin of Fenfluramine (Pondimin). What made Redux a new and improved diet pill was its increased efficacy at decreasing hunger sensation, thus improving overall weight loss success. Like its first-generation cousin Pondimin, Redux works on the brain chemical called serotonin (see earlier in chapter) primarily by preventing the re-uptake and subsequent breakdown of serotonin. This process leads to an increased level of serotonin in the brain with a subsequent decrease in appetite and ultimately, a lower calorie intake.

Redux, available by prescription only, was never recommended for cosmetic weight loss. It was indicated only for obese patients with an initial body mass index (BMI) of at least 30 (approximately 30 percent above the healthy weight range) or a BMI of at least 27 (approximately 20 percent above the healthy weight range) in the presence of other risk factors such as hypertension or high cholesterol.

Redux Update

Recent health concerns by leading physicians and weight loss experts regarding Redux and fenfluramine have led to the withdrawing of these two drugs from pharmacy shelves.

The recall in September 1997 of both dexfenfluramine (Redux) and fenfluramine (Pondimin) from the marketplace seems shocking at first, but less so after some of the facts are known.

Initial approval of Redux by the Food and Drug Administration's (FDA) specially appointed advisory panel did not happen without a lot of controversy. When the advisory panel convened back in September 1995, the data presented on Redux by Interneuron Pharmaceuticals, Inc., the drug company responsible for distributing Redux worldwide, seemed indisputable: Redux worked! Over 60 million people in Europe and elsewhere in the world had used Redux for treating obesity since the mid 1980s. The panel had no trouble seeing the positive aspects of Redux's weight loss capabilities and voted overwhelmingly to affirm the effectiveness of the drug.

Problems began when information on side effects and serious complications related to the use of Redux were addressed. In September 1995, the FDA-appointed advisory panel knew only that Redux was linked to a rare but fatal condition known as Primary Pulmonary Hypertension (PPH). On its own, PPH is a rare occurrence in the general population, affecting one or two out of a million people. Symptoms of PPH include shortness of breath, fainting, chest pain and swelling of the legs,

Data accumulated during the 1980s on the use of Redux in Europe and the rest of the world showed that taking Redux increased one's chances of developing PPH to roughly 18 per million. Additionally, laboratory studies appeared to demonstrate evidence of brain damage in several animals given Redux.

The panel also addressed the issue of whether Redux was safe for long-term use. After considering research findings, the panel decided not to delay the entry of Redux into the marketplace, even though long-term studies in North America were lacking. The impact of obesity on the health of Americans was thought by the FDA to be too devastating not to grant approval of Redux. The panel approved Redux by a vote of 6 to 5 in November 1995. It was agreed that long-term studies would be continued, this time collecting data on US citizens.

April 1996 heralded the availability of Redux, the first weight loss drug approved for public use by the FDA in twenty-three years. Ironically, the last weight loss drug to receive FDA approval was fenfluramine (Redux's older cousin) back in 1973.

Since its introduction, Redux has been taken by millions of North Americans in their quest for thinner and trimmer bodies.

Later in 1996, the year the drug was launched in the US, new data from Europe on complications related to the use of Redux were released. The risk of developing PPH was not 18 per million, but 23 to 46 per million! Still, Redux continued to be prescribed in record numbers.

Only in 1997 was heart valve disease linked with taking Redux or Pondimin. In July 1997, physicians at the Mayo Clinic in Rochester, Minnesota, reported a trend: 24 new cases of heart problems related to taking these diet pills. At about the same time, a 29-year-old woman in Boston died of PPH, and it was learned that she had been taking Fen-Phen.

In September 1997, the FDA completed its own analysis of the most recent data. Their conclusion: taking Redux or Pondimin caused worrisome heart valve abnormalities in 32 percent of the 291 patients across the US who were included in the study. These heart problems, which can be detected by a cardiologist or a trained technician doing an echocardiogram (ultrasound of the heart), are potentially dangerous to one's health. Thickened heart valves seen in affected patients can lead to a higher risk of heart failure because the condition imposes a heavier work load on the heart.

Dr. Sam's Views on Redux

Redux was part of the comprehensive weight-loss plan I offered my patients who met the weight criteria.

My patients were informed of both major and minor side effects of taking these "magic pills," and we reached a conclusion about the relative risk and benefits for each Redux candidate before I put pen to paper to write the prescription.

My patients were then monitored carefully during their treatment period. Their heart and lungs were examined each time they came to my office for their follow-up visits. Of all my patients who took Redux, those who did exceptionally well were the ones who also made changes in their lifestyle. These successful people incorporated exercise, a change in eating habits and a whole new attitude toward food into their lives. These are the people who did well on Redux.

New Pills on the Horizon

The search for a magic pill goes on. Researchers are as busy as ever in their work to uncover a possibly unknown mechanism in the human body that turns our "thin genes" on and our "fat genes" off. You will be reading more about obesity genes in the future as scientists and researchers try to uncover the few secrets of life that are still unknown to mankind.

Prescribing weight-loss pills is a choice all medical doctors must make when dealing with a seriously obese patient who desperately needs to lose weight—or die!

Addendum

Several new medications are currently being considered by the Food and Drug Administration or by the manufacturer for public use.

Phen-Pro is a new weight-loss combination of two FDA-approved drugs, Phentermine and Prozac. However, Prozac has not been specifically approved by the FDA for weight loss treatment. Experts and regulators have yet to pass judgment on the advisability of this new combination of medications to lose weight.

Sibutramine (Meridia). This medication uses a dual mechanism: 1) increasing serotonin function in the brain and 2) increasing norepinephrine brain levels. Side effects of hypertension (even though occurring in only 1 percent of the test population) may raise concern about its use.

Orlistat (Xenical). Xenical works by decreasing fat absorption in the intestines, leading to increased excretion of fat in the stool. Xenical was shown to increase weight loss by 16 percent over placebos in studies lasting two years. Side effects, such as soft stools and decreased absorption of vitamin D and other nutrients, can occur. Its approval for the public's use has been delayed over the manufacturer's concern of a possible link between Xenical and breast cancer.

The news isn't full of glory, though. To you, my reader, I end this section with the hope that you realize there is no magic pill to ward off obesity. The effectiveness of any weight-loss pill will be enhanced by learning healthier eating habits as well as by incorporating exercise into your lifestyle. Don't be shy to share your concerns with your doctor or trusted health care provider. But remember: *caveat emptor* (buyer beware)!

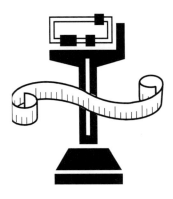

Chapter 16

"Wonder" Diets

FOR A LONG TIME I HAVE WONDERED, "What exactly is a wonder diet?" Even more basic, I have been intrigued by our global use of the word: **diet**. According to the *Webster's International Collegiate Dictionary*, the word "diet" is defined as a) the food and drink that a person, animal, or group usually consumes; b) the kind and amount of food selected for a person or animal for a special reason (as in ill health or obesity); c) something provided especially habitually (as in a steady diet of television); d) to eat or cause to eat less according to a set of rules; or finally, e) a formal deliberative assembly (e.g. a governmental legislative assembly). For our purposes here, we will consider definitions a, b, and d.

Where did the word "diet" come from? As do most words, the word "diet" originates from one or more of our ancestral languages: from Old French (*diete*), Latin (*diaeta*, meaning "prescribed diet"), or Greek (*diaita*, literally "manner of living"). One can argue that diet has its roots in the word *dies*, Latin for "day"!

When we use the word "diet," we are generally referring to our day's meal or menu plan. If you are one of the over 40 million Americans who are currently on some sort of a "diet," you know that the word has achieved a level of notoriety. This now infamous word reverberates with negative vibrations when spoken by fellow dieters. The reason is clear: diets imply deprivation! It is no wonder people cringe when the "D-word" is brought up in casual conversation. "What diet are you on now?" we often hear people asking each other. One of our favorite bashing words of the 1990s is **diet**!

I'm here to change all that! I want to change all of our learned responses to the now ugly and much maligned word, "diet."

I need your help to accomplish this seemingly monumental but most important task. We don't have to learn to hate the "D-word" if we can replace the word "diet" with a better, more user-friendly expression in our daily reference to our eating habits.

Expressions such as "menu plan" or "meal plan" conjure up much better feelings and less restrictive and constricting images than the word "diet." I would rather hear my patients telling me, "Gee, doc. I tried that new menu plan you suggested and not only did I lose weight, but I feel great. Thanks."

Doesn't that sound more encouraging and less evocative of a boring, barely bearable attitude that is so widespread when talking about a "diet?"

Of course, one could always develop a new word to replace the old and tired word, "diet." Acronyms come to mind. For example, when plannings your day's menu, you want to maximize your "Healthy Eating And Drinking Intake." Your "HEADI" would be full of healthful food and drink for your body. Or you could prepare your daily "Balanced Nutritional System" and call it BANUSY.

"Wonder" Diets

Here for your amusement are some of the "wonder diets" that have come and gone over the years. See if you recognize any of them that you may have tried. These "wonder diets" are certainly no panacea to our society's obesity troubles. They do, however, provide plenty of "food" for thought! Remember: **DIETS DON'T WORK!**

- ✔ Atkins Diet
- ✔ All You Can Eat Diet (the favorite)
- ✔ Bean Sprout Diet
- ✔ Beverly Hills Diet
- ✔ Cabbage Diet
- ✔ Carbohydrate Craver's Diet
- ✔ The California Diet
- ✔ The F-Plan
- ✔ Grapefruit Diet
- ✔ I Love America Diet
- ✔ I Love New York Diet
- ✔ Jack Sprat Diet
- ✔ Pritikin Diet
- ✔ Religious Diet
- ✔ Richard Simmons Diet
- ✔ Scarsdale Diet
- ✔ Stillman Diet
- ✔ Duct Tape Diet
- ✔ The Mayo Clinic Diet

The list goes on!

Diets don't work because they do not address lifestyle change. Most people find it very difficult to commit to a permanent change in lifestyle. Instead, it is easier to undergo a brief, temporary, and usually intense period of deprivation to achieve a desired short-term weight-loss goal. Once the diet is over, people revert to their old ways of eating—and gain weight. No wonder diets don't work!

Most diets do not provide an adequate supply of the nutrients your body needs to stay healthy, especially the right proportion of vitamins and minerals. As a result, dieters are required to take vitamin and mineral supplements in order to maintain nutritional balance. More often than not, these supplements end up becoming substitutes for the right food, a much less desirable outcome. No wonder that diets are temporary, and therefore doomed to fail.

Do you think that vitamin supplements are good for you? Ask yourself if you know exactly what goes into a vitamin pill. Wouldn't it be more enjoyable to bite into a juicy, ripe peach or take a bite out of a solid, red delicious apple than pop a boring and unappetizing vitamin pill? Still skeptical about believing that vitamin pills are inferior to the real thing? Listen to the experts. Here is a statement taken from a 1995 issue of the *Journal of American Medical Association* (paraphrased and shortened here for brevity) signed by 18 leading nutrition researchers and medical authorities commenting on food vs. vitamin pills:

> A growing body of research evidence indicates that vitamin pills—even in adequate amounts—do not offer the full complement of nutrients provided by food. Along with the vitamins in food come fiber and calories, which are necessary at all ages. In addition, food provides the perfect medium for the proper absorption and distribution of vitamins for

bodily needs. Nutrients are best absorbed from foods where they interact with other food ingredients. Vitamins in pure or concentrated form are more likely to interfere with each other's absorption, or with the absorption of nutrients in foods eaten at the same time. It is not uncommon to find cases wherein concentrated vitamin supplements produce toxic reactions in the body.

Conclusion: Good food is better than good pills.

I hope you are now convinced that no matter how many "diets" you may try, the best diet is no diet at all. That's right! For maximum health and best results from your body, you need to feed your greatest asset a regular amount and a wide variety of healthy foods from all five food groups. (See Chapter 4, "Back to Basics: The Food Guide Pyramid.")

As you can see in the list of diets on the preceding pages, the overwhelming majority of what we call "diets" are formulated for weight loss. Some diets claim to work immediately on your excess weight; others may take a little persistence and patience. What most people learn from a diet is to ask one question: "When is this diet over?"

"What do you think of diets, Sophie? Don't you think that the word 'diet,' with its negative connotation, should be replaced, or dare I say it, removed from our daily conversation?"

"I agree with you that there have been too many weight-loss diets promising instant health, perfectly toned bodies, and almost everything else, including fame and fortune. No diet will ever do that! You're right, Sam. The word 'diet' evokes feelings of deprivation in people who are trying to lose weight.

"Diets do have their place in the treatment of medical conditions, some of which are anemia, hypertension, and diabetes. However, for most relatively healthy individuals who wish to lose weight, following a 'diet' does not guarantee long-term success."

"What do you recommend instead of diets?"

"I encourage my clients to listen to their bodies. This means knowing when you first feel hunger. It could be the faintest empty feeling in your stomach, or perhaps a let-down in your energy level. Whatever the clue, feeling hungry is an individual sensation."

"What does being aware of when you're feeling hungry have to do with losing weight?"

"Since I do not direct my clients to follow a weight-reducing diet, I teach them instead to monitor their hunger by using **"The Hunger Scale."** Using this scale, they will learn to recognize their particular hunger pattern.

"I'm intrigued. Please explain your scale."

"Certainly. It's very simple. A diagram here will help:

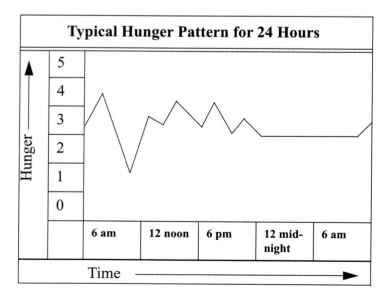

"Wonder" Diets

"The first diagram, known as the 'Typical Hunger Pattern' shows hunger plotted against time of day. As shown on this chart, there are customary times throughout the day when people tend to get hungrier. These times usually precede their meals. Each of my clients is given an assignment to complete before their second consultation with me. I ask them to rate their hunger every hour on a scale of 0 to 5 throughout one waking day, with 0 representing no hunger and 5 representing maximum hunger. The results are brought back to me at the next visit for discussion."

"What kind of results do you usually see?"

"Most people fall into one of two categories. The first category is illustrated in the following diagram known as the 'Overeaters' Hunger Pattern.'"

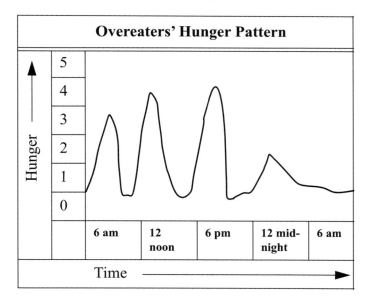

"This pattern is typical for most North Americans who overeat at mealtimes. They feel ravenously hungry before meals, eat until they are completely satiated, then wait until they are again extremely hungry before eating their next meal. This pattern I call the 'Icicle' because of the sharp, intense peaks of hunger experienced by people in this category."

"What about the other common category of people you see?"

"Look at the following diagram. This pattern reveals to me that the person within this category never truly feels hungry, yet eats anyway to stave off any true feeling of hunger. Snacking is also rampant within this category. This type of eating pattern generally signifies a fear of hunger. Therefore, I call this the 'Fear of Hunger' pattern."

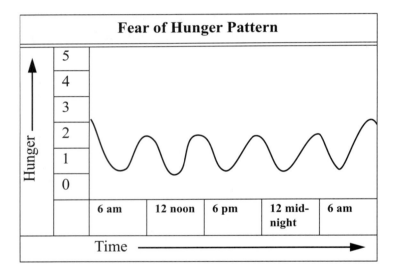

"Are there any other patterns you come across in dealing with your clients?"

"Yes. I also see patterns that indicate eating disorders such as bulimia or anorexia nervosa.

"With all of my clients, the goal is to reduce the wide fluctuations in their hunger."

"In other words, you want your clients to know when and how hungry they are so that their hunger patterns look like the two following patterns."

"Right, Sam. The first desirable pattern (A) demonstrates eating within the 'comfort zone' of hunger and fullness. This pattern is achieved by eating three small meals and two to three snacks a day. The second pattern (B) displays an eating pattern with more frequent snacks and smaller meals. This is ideal for weight loss and subsequent weight control. This eating pattern is well known by its alternate name: GRAZING." (See Chapter 3, "Time to Eat.")

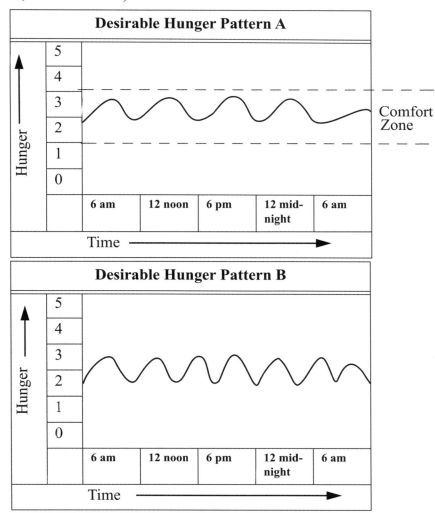

The End of Obesity

"Thanks for the information on hunger scales and the impact of hunger on eating patterns. I would like to return to the idea of diets for a moment. You know, Sophie, there are several new ways people are trying to lose weight and keep it off. For example, I read an ad in a popular magazine about how weight loss can be achieved through reflexology!"

"Tell me more."

"A doctor in Europe claims that by wearing a special insole in your shoe, you will stimulate your digestive organs to burn excess fat."

"Amazing! Why haven't I heard of this?"

"Probably because it will never get off the ground. All talk and no action!"

"I do consider reflexology, the belief that all of the body's organs have a reflex point somewhere on the soles of the feet, to have some merit. I know I feel relaxed when you rub my feet. However, walking, no matter what shoes are worn, will help speed up a person's metabolism."

"I have also heard about aromatherapy for weight loss. The approach is as follows: inhale a particular blend of scents while holding the tempting food next to your mouth. According to the advertisers, the smell that will now be associated with this food will no longer be appetizing. Thus, you will no longer crave that food."

"What will people think of next?"

"The weight-loss industry is a multi-billion dollar one, and people want in. Americans spent more than sixty billion dollars on weight-loss products in 1996! The way I see it, our only defense against the proliferation of all these ridiculous and potentially dangerous weight-loss schemes is educating people with correct information. That's why we are here right now discussing all of the above. Ignorance may be bliss, but knowledge is power."

"I agree."

"Wonder" Diets

"Sophie, there is one other method of weight control that we have not talked about, but that deserves mention. It is the preferred way of keeping weight off for millions of people in North America, mostly in the young adult and adolescent population."

"Are you referring to binging and purging?"

"No, not at the moment. I'm talking about the most disgusting and lethal habit that has invaded our society for the last three and a half centuries, but more so since the beginning of the twentieth century. It is an addiction that is widely promoted as 'cool' and 'hip' by their producers. There is no doubt in my mind that cigarettes, or 'cancer sticks,' are the tried and true method of weight loss and weight control for many teenagers and others in the latter part of this century."

"You have a point. Just open any women's magazine these days and you'll see cigarette ads depicting a tall, slender and sophisticated-looking woman engaging in an interesting and lively activity while she is holding her lit cigarette. The message being conveyed is as plain as the beauty mark on your cheek, Sam: Cigarettes make you look healthy and slim and help keep you at your ideal weight."

"That's what the tobacco industry wants America's youth to believe. The nicotine in each cigarette is a powerful drug. Its mechanism of action in the brain is so diverse and its hold on the smoker is so gripping that it is no wonder that cigarette smoking is considered by many experts to be the most difficult drug addiction to give up.

"As with all addicting substances, nicotine stimulates certain receptors within the brain, leading to an overall sense of well-being. Each puff from a cigarette positively reinforces this pleasurable sensation. Going without a cigarette for several hours leads to the unpleasant feeling of withdrawal, including impatience and irritability, a general sense of malaise and fatigue, decreased alertness and concentration, and most of all, an increase in appetite and potential weight gain. For all of the above reasons, and many more, the smoker finds it extremely difficult to quit smoking."

"How do you encourage your smoking patients to quit?"

"First, I inquire if they have ever tried to quit smoking, or if they are planning to quit in the near future. I then advise them on the benefits of quitting smoking. When my patients are adolescents, I know that talking about long-term health problems such as lung cancer, emphysema, heart attacks, and other later-in-life diseases do not scare them. Teenagers need to be told that smoking is unattractive, smelly, stinky, and not the cool thing they think it is. Bad breath, yellow teeth, and decreased athletic performance may sway our youth to believe that smoking is not for them.

"The pricing policy of cigarettes is another problem. A pack of cigarettes should not be sold for the price of candy. Poison should not be made so readily available to our children and at such low prices as we see in most stores where tobacco products are sold. No tobacco products should be sold to minors—period. One puff from a cigarette is one puff too many.

"There is no good reason to experiment with smoking cigarettes, especially not, 'because everyone else is doing it.' The gain might be temporary popularity, but the losses are bad health, a lack of control over your body, and a lifetime of dependence on nicotine products, with an almost certain sickly existence in the second half of your life. Are cigarettes worth it?

"I know first-hand how smoking can ruin a person's health and bring heartache to a family.

"My father smoked for over a decade in his younger years. Fortunately, he quit when he married my mother. But he worked with people who smoked. I recall every day my father returning home from work and reeking of smoke. Back then, I thought that the smell of smoke was normal at the workplace since my father's suits were so full of that smoky smell.

"My dad's luck ran out when he turned fifty. After inhaling that noxious second-hand smoke for so many years, dad developed a nagging cough that would not go away. He went to see his doctor. An exam and a chest X-ray confirmed the worst: my father had lung cancer. He died four months later, after suffering through several rounds of chemotherapy and its humiliating effects.

"My father died because he smoked and because he spent most of his life breathing the smoke of other smokers. As a doctor, I'm here to help prevent as many people as possible from experiencing the terrible fate that befell my father. I've told my father's story many times. Somehow it gives meaning to his death.

"I need some help from you, Sophie. Can you think of ways to help people avoid the munchies and subsequent weight gain that seems inevitable when people stop smoking?"

"That's what this book is all about: taming and conquering obesity. Many people tell me that they were satisfied with their weight until they gave up cigarettes. Then their weight ballooned anywhere from ten to one hundred pounds after they kicked their cigarette habit.

"Part of the reason why people gain weight after quitting smoking is that the movement of hand to mouth associated with smoking is difficult to forget. Unlearning this habitual movement takes time. During this unlearning period, it is top priority for recent quitters to surround themselves with the most low-fat, low-calorie foods available.

"The appetite-suppressing effect of nicotine is gone, and the urge to eat and put something in the mouth is that much stronger. The result can be a tremendous weight gain in a very short period of time.

"I have devised a series of suggestions for recently liberated ex-smokers that can help them through the one to four weeks of highest risk of potential weight gain.

1. Stay out of the kitchen!

As a smoker goes about getting rid of the cigarette habit, there will be intense cravings not just for the cigarette but for literally anything to be placed in the mouth as a form of comfort. Food is the number one comfort item of all new ex-smokers.

Easily eaten and swallowed foods, such as candy bars, donuts, and anything that is sweet, soft and chewy, are the preferred food items of people who are quitting smoking. The problem is that repeated hand-to-mouth action leads to overconsumption of calories due to an improper choice of foods as well as from an increase in amount eaten. There is only one way to avoid this phenomenon which invariably results in a significant weight gain: do something else.

Alternate activities should take place outside of the kitchen and be interesting enough to distract you from both smoking and eating. Good home activities include sewing, cleaning the house, writing, using the computer, talking with a non-smoker, even singing.

Outdoor activities are even better as they get you away from household cues for smoking and eating. Biking, mowing the lawn, shoveling snow, walking with a friend, playing with your children are excellent outdoor activities to keep you from cigarettes.

You can probably think of dozens of other activities you can do in order to distract yourself from your food and cigarette cravings. (See Chapter 9: "Mood for Food.")

"Wonder" Diets

2. If you decide to give in to your food cravings, have the right foods ready for eating.

Many of my clients like crunching on baby carrots. Other fresh vegetables can be cut ahead of time and placed in the refrigerator, ready for times when you need to put some food in your mouth. Fresh veggies such as green, red, or yellow peppers, cucumbers, celery, cauliflower, and broccoli provide very few calories compared to one cream-filled pastry or one chocolate-coated candy bar!

3. Don't tempt yourself.

Here are some helpful hints that you can use in the kitchen or elsewhere to lessen your chances of unnecessary nibbling while beating the smoking habit:

- ✔ Keep cookies and other sweets in opaque rather than see-through containers to keep yourself from strong visual reminders of the temptation inside.

- ✔ Store high-calorie, high-fat foods on hard to reach shelves in your pantry. For refrigerator items, store these foods in the back part of the lower shelves, out of easy reach.

- ✔ Store low-calorie foods so that they are readily available and visible.

- ✔ Move non-food activities, such as paying bills at the kitchen table, out of the kitchen and away from temptation.

- ✔ Don't store candy and nuts in dishes throughout the house, especially in the den or living room where they are too accessible and too easy to pick at.

✔ During your coffee break, try doing something other than eating. Walk around the block or run a quick errand.

✔ When attending parties, have a healthy snack before going. This helps to reduce your risk of overindulging in your favorite munchies.

You can come up with many more ideas. All it takes is a little creativity and perseverance.

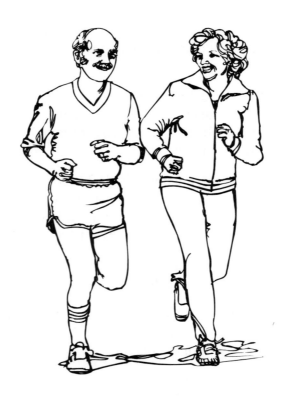

Your Turn

SOPHIE AND I HAVE ENJOYED presenting to you some of the insights we've gained through the years from our patients, clients, friends—and from each other.

No matter how wise you become in the way your marvelous human body functions, no matter how much knowledge you accumulate about the role of good nutrition and exercise in building a healthy body, no matter how clearly you understand biochemical reactions or the intricacies of the digestive system, it won't do anything for you personally until you start putting principles of healthful living into practice in your daily life.

Today is not too late. In fact, today is the best time in all the world for you to begin.

Make nature's finest and simplest foods the mainstay of your diet. Learn the signals your body gives you when it's really hungry. Let yourself thoroughly enjoy food and exercise. Have fun living healthfully!

Too many people are burdened by a haunting fear of obesity and end up trapped in the very habits that lead to overweight and poor muscle tone. You don't have to be one of those unfortunate people. Now you know how to be free from worries about what you eat and how much you weigh. You can look it in the face and know that for the rest of your life you have seen—

The End of Obesity.

Recommended Reading

We have compiled a short but interesting reading list that we feel complements our book's ideas and recommendations. Happy reading (and eating)!

1. Bailey, Lee (1966). *Portable Food.* New York, New York: Clarkson N. Potter, Inc.

2. Clark, Nancy, M.S., R.D. (1996). *Sports Nutrition Guidebook, Second Ed.*, Champagne, IL: Human Kinetics Publishers.

3. Goldbeck, Niki & Davie (1992). *The Good Breakfast Book.* Woodstock, New York: Ceres Press.

4. Grundy, Scott M., M.D., Ph.D.; Mary Winston, Ed.D., R.D. (1989). *The American Heart Association Low-Fat, Low-Cholesterol Cookbook.* New York, New York: Times Books.

5. Katzen, Mollie (1992). *Moosewood Cookbook.* Berkeley, California: Ten Speed Press.

6. Larson Duyff, Robeta (1996). *The American Dietetic Association's Complete Food & Nutrition Guide.* Minneapolis, Minnesota: Chronimed Publishing.

7. McDonald, Arline, Ph.D., R.D.; Annette Natow, Ph.D., R.D.; Jo-Ann Heslin, M.S., R.D. (1994). *Complete Book of Vitamins and Minerals.* Publications International, Ltd.

8. Nissenberg, Sandra, M.S., R.D. et al (1995), *Quick Meals for Healthy Kids and Busy Parents.* Minnetonka, Minnesota: Chronimed Publishing.

9. Peck, Carole (1997). *The Buffet Book.* New York, New York: The Penguin Group.

10. Pytka, Evelyne (1993). *Almonds & Raisins and Mostly Muffins.* Montreal, Canada: Evelyne Pytka.

11. Robertson, Laurel, Carol Flinders, Bronwen Godfrey, (1982). *Laurel's Kitchen.* Petaluma, California: Nilgiri Press.

12. Schwartz, Rosie (1989). *The Enlightened Eater.* Toronto, Canada: Stoddart Publishing Co., Ltd.

13. Smith, M.J., M.A., R.D., (1997). *All-American Low-Fat Meals in Minutes.* Minneapolis, Minnesota: Chronimed Publishing.

14. Sullivan, Karen (1997). *Vitamins & Minerals.* Brisbane, Australia: Element Books., Ltd.

15. Williams, Sallie Y. (1995). *Vegetables on the Side.* New York, New York: Simon & Schuster Macmillan Company.

Order Form

Please send ___ copies of *The End of Obesity* **at US $14.95 each plus $3.00 shipping and handling to:**

Name:_____

Address: _____

City:_____State:___ Zip:_____

Mail this order form to:
    G&G Publishing
    379 Amherst St.
    Nashua, NH 03063

Make your check or money order payable to G&G Publishing.

Discount available for orders of 5 or more books to one address. Call 603 594-0986 for rates.

Order Form

Please send ___ copies of *The End of Obesity* **at US $14.95 each plus $3.00 shipping and handling to:**

Name:_____

Address: _____

City:_____State:___ Zip:_____

Mail this order form to:
    G&G Publishing
    379 Amherst St.
    Nashua, NH 03063

Make your check or money order payable to G&G Publishing.

Discount available for orders of 5 or more books to one address. Call 603 594-0986 for rates.